RENAL DIET

MW01047625

150+ Easy and Delicious Recipes to Control Your Kidney Disease and Avoid Dialysis. Only Low Sodium, Low Potassium, Low Phosphorus and Healthy Recipes

© Jaida Ellison

Legal & Disclaimer

TABLE OF CONTENTS

INTRODUCTION

Human health hangs in a complete balance when all of its interconnected bodily mechanisms function properly in perfect sync. Without its major organs working normally, the body soon suffers indelible damage. Kidney malfunction is one such example, and it is not just the entire water balance that is disturbed by the kidney disease, but a number of other diseases also emerge due to this problem. Kidney diseases are progressive in nature, meaning that if left unchecked and uncontrolled, they can ultimately lead to permanent kidney damage. That is why it is essential to control and manage the disease and put a halt to its progress, which can be done through medicinal and natural means. While medicines can guarantee only thirty percent of the cure, a change of lifestyle and diet can prove to be miraculous with their seventy percent of guaranteed results. A kidney-friendly diet and lifestyle not only saves the kidneys from excess minerals, but it also aids medicines to work actively. Treatment without a good diet, hence, proves to be useless. In this renal diet cookbook, we shall bring out the basic facts about kidney diseases, their symptoms, causes, and diagnosis. This preliminary introduction can help the readers understand the problem clearly; then, we shall discuss the role of renal diet and kidney-friendly lifestyle in curbing the diseases. And it's not just that, the book also contains a range of delicious renal diet recipes which will guarantee luscious flavors and good health.

CHAPTER 1:
Understanding kidney disease

Before stepping further into the depths of the renal diet, let us learn more about our kidneys and how they function. This basic understanding can ensure a better awareness of kidney disease. Our kidneys act just like a filter; in fact, they are the natural filter of the body, which mainly filters the blood running into them with high pressure. There is one kidney on either side of the body; they both work in sync to clean and purify the entire body's blood constantly and consistently. The renal arteries that enter the kidneys also pass by the membranes in it, which only let the harmful excretory products to pass into the ureters of the kidneys and render the blood cleaned and purified. There is another vital function that the kidneys play which is to keep the water and electrolyte balance maintained in the body. If our body has water in excess, the kidneys will release it through urination, and if our body is dehydrated, then more water is retained. This smart mechanism is only possible when a critical mineral balance is maintained inside the kidney cells since the release of water can only occur through osmosis.

Kidney function or renal function are the terms used to explain how well the kidneys function. A healthy individual is born with a pair of kidneys. This is why whenever one of the kidneys lost its functioning it went unnoticed due to the function of the other kidney. But if the kidney functions further drop altogether and reach a level as low as 25 percent, it turns out to be serious for the patients. People who have only one kidney functioning need proper external therapy and in worst cases, a kidney transplant.

Kidney diseases occur when a number of renal cells known as nephrons are either partially or completely damaged and fail to properly filter blood entering in. The gradual damage of the kidney cells can occur due to various reasons, sometimes it is the acidic or toxic build-up inside the kidney over time, at times it is genetic, or the result of other kidney damaging diseases like hypertension (high blood pressure) or diabetes.

Chronic Kidney Disease (CKD)

CKD or chronic kidney disease is the stage of kidney damage where it fails to filter the blood properly. The term chronic is used to refer to gradual and long-term damage to an organ. Chronic kidney disease is therefore developed after a slow yet progressive damage to the kidneys. The symptoms of this disease only appear when the toxic wastes start to build up in the body. Therefore, such a stage should be prevented at all costs. Hence, early diagnosis of the disease proves to be significant. The sooner the patient realizes the gravity of the situation, the better measures he can take to curb the problem.

What are the causes of kidney disease?

There is never a single cause for a disease; a number of factors come into play and together become the source of the renal deficiency. As stated earlier, these causes may include the genetics of a person, some other health disorders that may damage the kidneys and the kind of lifestyle a person lives. The following are the most commonly known causes of renal disease.

- Heart disease
- Diabetes
- Hypertension (High blood pressure)
- Being around 60 years old
- Having kidney disease in family

Signs of renal disease

The good thing is that we can prevent the chronic stage of renal disease by identifying the early signs of any form of kidney damage. Even when a person feels minor changes in his body, he should consult an expert to confirm if it might lead to something serious. The following are a few of the early symptoms of renal damage:

- Tiredness or drowsiness
- Muscle cramps
- Loss of appetite

- Changes in the frequency of urination
- Swelling of hands and feet
- A feeling of itchiness
- Numbness
- The darkness of skin
- Trouble in sleeping
- Shortness of breath
- The feeling of nausea or vomiting

These symptoms can appear in combination with one another. These are general signs of body malfunction, and they should never be ignored. And if they are left unnoticed, they can lead to worsening of the condition and may appear as:

- Back pain
- Abdominal pain
- Fever
- Rash
- Diarrhea
- Nosebleeds
- Vomiting

After witnessing any of these symptoms, a person should immediately consult a health expert and prepare himself or herself for the required lifestyle changes.

Stages of renal disease

According to the National Kidney Foundation in the US, kidney disease can be classified into five different progressive stages. These stages and their symptoms do not only help the doctor to devise an appropriate therapy but also guide the patient to take the necessary measures in routine life. The rate of kidney function actually tells much about these phases. In the early stages, there is minimum loss of function, and this loss increases with every stage.

The eGFR is used as a standard criterion to measure the Kidney function. eGFR is the acronym for the estimated Glomerular Filtration Rate. It is the rate at which the waste material is transferred from the blood to the nephron's tubes through "glomerulus"- the filtering membrane of the kidney tissues. The lesser the rate of glomerular filtration, the greater the problem the kidneys are going through. A person's age, gender, race, and serum creatinine are entered into a mathematical formula to calculate his eGFR. The serum creatinine level is measured in a blood test. The creatinine is actually a waste product of the body which is produced out of muscular activities. Healthy kidneys are capable of removing all the creatinine out of the blood. A rising creatinine level is therefore a sign of kidney disease. It is said that if a person has been having an eGFR of less than 60 for three months, it means that he is suffering from serious renal problems.

The five main stages of chronic kidney disease can be categorized as follows:

- Stage 1:

The first stage starts when the eGFR gets slightly higher than the normal value. In this stage, the eGFR can be equal or greater than 90mL/min

- Stage 2:

The next stage arises when the eGFR starts to decline and ranges between 60 to 89 mL/min. It is best to control the progression of the disease at this point.

- Stage 3:

From this point on, the kidney disease becomes concerning for the patient as the eGFR drops to 30-59 mL/min. At this stage, consultation is essential for the health of the patient.

- Stage 4:

The stage 4 is also known as Severe Chronic Kidney Diseases as the eGFR level drops to 15-29 mL/min.

- Stage 5:

The final and most critical phase of chronic renal disease is stage 5, where the estimated glomerular filtration rate gets as low as below 15 mL/min.

Renal disease diagnostic tests

Besides identifying the symptoms of kidney disease, there are other better and more accurate ways to confirm the extent of loss of renal function. There are mainly two important diagnostic tests:

1. Urine test

The urine test clearly states all the renal problems. The urine is the waste product of the kidney. When there is loss of filtration or any hindrance to the kidneys, the urine sample will indicate it through the number of excretory products present in it. The severe stages of chronic disease show some amount of protein and blood in the urine. Do not rely on self-tests; visit an authentic clinic for these tests.

2. Blood pressure and blood test

Another good way to check for renal disease is to test the blood and its composition. A high amount of creatinine and other waste products in the blood clearly indicates that the kidneys are not functioning properly. Blood pressure can also be indicative of renal disease. When the water balance in the body is disturbed, it may cause high blood pressure. Hypertension can both be the cause and symptom of kidney disease and therefore should be taken seriously.

How to keep your kidneys healthy

Like all other parts of the body, human kidneys also need much care and attention to work effectively. It takes a few simple and consistent measures to keep them healthy. Remember that no medicine can guarantee good health, but only a better lifestyle can do so. Here are a few of the practices that can keep your kidneys stay healthy for life.

1. Active lifestyle

An active routine is imperative for good health. This may include regular exercise, yoga, or sports and physical activities. The more you move your body, the better its metabolism gets. The loss of water is compensated by drinking more water, and that constantly drains all the toxins and waste from the kidneys. It also helps in controlling blood pressure, cholesterol levels, and diabetes, which indirectly prevents kidney disease.

2. Control blood pressure

Constant high blood pressure may cause glomerular damage. It is one of the leading causes, and every 3 out of 5 people suffering from hypertension also suffer from kidney problems. The normal human blood pressure is below 120/80 mmHg. When there is a constant increase of this pressure up to 140/100mmHg or more it should be immediately put under control. This can be done by minimizing the salt intake, controlling the cholesterol level and taking care of cardiac health.

3. Hydration

Drinking more water and salt-free fluids proves to be the life support for kidneys. Water and fluids dilute the blood consistency and lead to more urination; this in turn will release most of the excretions out of the body without much difficulty. Drinking at least eight glasses of water in a day is essential. It is basically the lack of water which strains the kidneys and often hinders the glomerular filtration. Water is the best option, but fresh fruit juices with no salt and preservatives are also vital for kidney health. Keep all of them in constant daily use.

4. Dietary changes

There are certain food items which taken in excess can cause renal problems. In this regard, an extremely high protein diet, food rich in sodium, potassium, and phosphorous can be harmful. People who are suffering from early stages of renal disease should reduce their intake, whereas those facing critical stages of CKD should avoid their use altogether. A well-planned renal diet can prove to be significant in this regard. It effectively restricts all such food items from the diet and promotes the use of more fluids, water, organic fruits, and a low protein meal plan.

5. No smoking/alcohol

Smoking and excessive use of alcohol are other names for intoxication. Intoxication is another major cause of kidney disease, or at least it aggravates the condition. Smoking and drinking alcohol indirectly pollute the blood and body tissues, which leads to progressive kidney damage. Begin by gradually reducing alcohol consumption and smoking down to a minimum.

6. Monitor the changes

Since the early signs of kidney disease are hardly detectable, it is important to keep track of the changes you witness in your body. Even the frequency of urination and loss of appetite are good enough reasons to be cautious and concerning. It is true that only a health expert can accurately diagnose the disease, but personal care and attention to minor changes is of key importance when it comes to CKD.

How to prevent dialysis naturally

Dialysis steps in as a last case scenario when both kidneys lose sufficient function to clean the blood. Before the toxicity reaches a damaging level, it must be eradicated through external sources. Individuals who suffer from acute kidney diseases end up going through dialysis to get their blood cleaned through the artificial dialysis machine. This dialysis machine mimics the role of our kidneys, and the blood is pumped into the machine, and then it is pumped back into the body simultaneously. People who never went through dialysis should know that it is one long and exhaustive process, which every renal patient hates to go through. Fortunately, there are some effective measures to avoid dialysis. This precautionary measure can stop the progression of renal disease and even cure it to some extent.

- Exercise regularly
- Don't smoke
- Avoid excess salt in your diet
- Control of diabetes
- Eat correctly and lose excess weight
- Control high blood pressure
- Talk with your health care team

Role of potassium, sodium, and phosphorous

1. SODIUM

Sodium is considered the most important electrolyte of the body next to chloride and potassium. The electrolytes are actually the substance that controls the flow of fluids into the cells and out of them. Sodium is mainly responsible for regulating blood volume and pressure. It is also involved in controlling muscle contraction and nerve functions. The acid-base balance in the blood and other body fluids is also regulated by sodium. Though sodium is important for the health and regulation of important body mechanisms, excessive sodium intake, especially when a person suffers from some stages of chronic kidney disease, can be dangerous. Excess sodium disrupts the critical fluid balance in the body and inside the kidneys. It then leads to high blood pressure, which in turn negatively affects the kidneys. Salt is one of the major sources of sodium in our diet, and it is strictly forbidden on the renal diet. High sodium intake can also lead to Edema, which is swelling of the face, hands, and legs. Furthermore, high blood pressure can stress the heart and cause the weakening of its muscles. The build-up of fluid in the lungs also leads to shortness of breath.

2. POTASSIUM

Potassium is another mineral that is closely linked to renal health. Potassium is another important electrolyte, so it maintains the fluid balance in the body and its pH levels as well. This electrolyte also plays an important role in controlling nerve impulses and muscular activity. It works in conjugation with the sodium to carry out all these functions. The normal potassium level in the blood must range between 3.5 and 5.5mEq/L. It is the kidneys that help maintain this balance, but without their proper function, the potassium starts to build up in the blood. Hyperkalemia is a condition characterized by high potassium levels. It usually occurs in people with chronic kidney disease. The prominent symptoms of high potassium are numbness, slow pulse rate, weakness, and nausea. Potassium is present in green vegetables and some fruits, and these ingredients should be avoided on a renal diet.

3. PHOSPHOROUS

The amount of phosphorus in the blood is largely linked to the functioning of the kidneys. Phosphorus, in combination with vitamin D, calcium, and parathyroid hormone, can regulate the renal function. The balance of phosphorous and calcium is maintained by the kidneys, and this balance keeps the bones and teeth healthy. Phosphorous, along with vitamin D, ensures the absorption of calcium into the bones and teeth, where this mineral is important for the body. On the other hand, it gets dangerous when the kidneys fail to control the amount of phosphorus in the blood. This may lead to heart and bone-related problems. Mainly there is a high risk of weakening of the bones followed by the hardening of the tissues due to the deposition of phosphorous and calcium outside the bones. This abnormal calcification can occur in the lungs, skin, joints, and arteries, which can become in time very painful. It may also result in bone pain and itching.

CHAPTER 2:
Kidney-friendly diet for healthier living

There is no denying of the fact that good food is equal to a healthy life. What makes good food is the control we have on our choices. The idea of empowered eating tells you how to consume food not just to satisfy your apparent appetite but also to fulfill all the nutritional, mental, and physical needs of your body. In this section, we shall seek the empowered eating by learning the dos and don'ts of the renal diet:

What to eat and drink and what to avoid in renal diet

All health-oriented diets follow a similar pattern: they all prescribe a restriction plan with some better dietary alternatives. By controlling the intake of certain food products, these diets can prove to be quite effective. To understand such diets, look into the what NOT to eat list, and the rest will be cleared on its own. So, here is what we are going to do: we shall break down the dos and don'ts of the renal diet and discuss the different food products that are safe or unsafe for the kidneys.

Lesser Sodium

As per the rules, a person must only consume less than 2300 mg of sodium per day in a renal diet. You see, sodium is the element that is present in all parts of the body and helps to maintain balance of fluid concentration. Too much sodium can, however, strain the kidney cells and eventually damage them as a result of the saturated internal environment. The question is, how can you avoid it? The answer is simple: cut off all high sodium products. Salt contains the most concentrated amount of sodium. So that needs to be avoided. Similarly, there are preserved, fermented, or processed food products that might contain sodium in a heavy amount; all such products should also be avoided.

There are several herbs or seasonings and even sauces like soy sauce that might contain a high dose of sodium, so either avoid them altogether or replace them with sodium-free products that are easily available in the market.

Ready-made soup powders, bouillon cubes, dips, broths, canned products, or fast food also have a high amount of sodium, and they should be avoided. In a nutshell, the following are items that you need to cross off from your renal diet grocery list:

- Salt of all types
- Fast food
- Processed food
- Brine dipped food

- Soy sauce and other high sodium sauces
- Fermented high sodium products
- Herbs and seasonings with sodium

Protein Intake

Proteins may not directly hurt or damage the kidney cells, yet when proteins are digested, they release uric acid or other toxic substances, which then are treated by the kidneys. The more abundant and complex these toxic by-products are, the harder the kidneys need to work, and in doing so, it might damage the kidneys' own cell due to toxicity. Normally red meat is prohibited to patients who suffer from high blood pressure and heart diseases. In the renal diet, a person should limit the intake of animal-based protein and try to get more of their proteins from white meat like poultry and seafood, such as the following.

Animal-protein foods:

- Chicken
- Eggs
- Fish
- Meat
- Dairy

When taken in small amounts per serving, these animal-based proteins will not strain the kidneys and will prevent damaging them. Two to three ounces of meat per serving and a half of cup yogurt, milk, or cheese per serving is enough to keep the kidneys healthy and burden-free.

Plant-protein foods:

- Nuts
- Beans
- Grains

Similarly, plant-based protein should be consumed in controlled proportions. Add a half of cup beans, a half of cup nuts per serving. Don't consume rice and noodles in quantities higher than a half of cup per serving.

Healthy Foods for Healthy Hearts

As stated earlier, the damage of the renal cells is largely due to constant high blood pressure. If we keep our heart healthy and control the blood pressure all the time, it will also be beneficial for the kidneys' health and functioning. To keep the heart healthy, we need to avoid foods with bad cholesterol and switch to foods with good cholesterol. The following food products should be consumed.

Heart-healthy foods:

- Beans
- Fruits
- Poultry without the skin

- Fish
- Vegetables
- Lean cuts of meat
- Low-fat or fat-free milk, yogurt, and cheese

Low Phosphorus Intake

Too much phosphorus in the blood can be dangerous as it can extract the calcium from the bones rendering them weak and thin. The decrease in calcium levels can also cause muscle tightness, spasms, itchy skin, and joint pain. All these symptoms are related to high levels of phosphorous. Many food products often contain this element, which is stated as PHOS on the labels. We should look for such items and avoid them. Down below are the lists of all the ingredients which are low in phosphorus, and these are highly recommended for the renal diet.

Foods with Low Phosphorus:

- Bread, pasta, rice
- Homemade iced tea
- Fresh fruits and vegetables
- Corn and rice cereals
- Rice milk (not enriched)
- Lemon/lime water
- Low phosphorous soda drinks

Foods with High Phosphorus:

- Meat, poultry, fish
- Bran cereals and oatmeal
- Soda drinks with phosphorous
- Dairy foods
- Canned iced tea
- Beans, lentils, nuts
- Canned or packed fruit juices, and punches

The list of foods higher in phosphorus shows the ingredients not suitable for a renal diet. Other than dietary changes, people can use phosphate binder to remove the phosphorous element while it is still in the stomach and release it from of the body without absorption.

The Right Amount of Potassium

Potassium in the right amount can keep the nerves and muscles working. Too low or too high of the potassium intake can cause health problems, including kidney damage and heart problems. Selecting the appropriate food products and controlling their intake keeps the potassium balanced in your body.

There are several salt-substitutes that provide heavy doses of potassium, so it is imperative to check the labels before buying. Also, check the labels of processed or canned vegetables and fruits to avoid excess potassium intake.

Foods with Low Potassium:

- Cooked carrots, green beans
- Apples, peaches
- White bread and pasta
- White rice
- Cooked rice and wheat cereals, grits
- Rice milk (not enriched)
- Apple, grape, or cranberry juice

Foods with High Potassium:

- Potatoes, tomatoes
- Bran cereals
- Dairy foods
- Beans and nuts
- Oranges, bananas, and orange juice
- Brown and wild rice
- Whole-wheat bread and pasta

Juices and Drinks Good for Renal Diet

The more organic natural and salt-free fluids we consume on a renal diet, the better it is for the kidneys. For kidney patients, consuming water in a good amount is essential. Try the following drinks and juices:

- Water
- Apple cider
- Cranberry juice cocktail

- Grape juice
- Lemonade

Fresh Fruit Juices

Extract fresh juices from the following fruits and blend them with water or ice. Drink juices regularly to increase your daily fluid intake.

- Apple
- Berries
- Cherries
- Fruit cocktail, drained
- Grapes
- Peach
- Pear, fresh or canned, drained
- Pineapple
- Plums
- Tangerine
- Watermelon

CHAPTER 3:
Frequently Asked Questions

Q1. How can we avoid phosphate additives in our kidney diet?

The practice of reading the labels can save you from all the trouble. It is not just the phosphates but a great number of other ingredients detrimental to a good renal diet that you can identify this way. When phosphate additives are present in the food, the label usually contains the E sign followed by a number showing the type of phosphate added to the product. Here is a list of commonly present phosphates in additives.

- E339 Sodium phosphates
- E338 Phosphoric acid
- E340 Potassium phosphates
- E343 Magnesium phosphates
- E545 Ammonium polyphosphates
- E450 Diphosphates
- E542 Bone phosphate
- E341 Calcium phosphates
- E540 Dicalcium diphosphate
- E541 Sodium aluminum phosphate
- E544 Calcium polyphosphates

Q2. What are the suitable alternatives to salt?

It is true that no spice and seasoning can replace salt, but when health comes first, we can make a little compromise on taste and try something that can infuse delicious flavors into our food even though not exactly like salt. Down below are a few examples that can be used to season beef, fish, pork, chicken and stews, etc.

1. For Beef, you can use dry mustard, allspice, bay leaf, oregano, chili powder, and cayenne pepper.

2. For the seasoning of the Fish, you can use lemon, vinegar, mint, dill, thyme, chili, garlic.

3. To spice up the Pork, you can use apple sauce, cloves, garlic powder, sage, onion powder, curry powder.

4. When it comes to Chicken and turkey, you can always use garlic, lemon, rosemary, thyme, chili powder, tarragon, sage, cayenne pepper, and paprika to season the meat.

5. For Stews and casseroles, try some sage, oregano, basil, thyme, and garlic to add flavors.

Q3. Is it safe to take herbal supplements on the Renal Diet?

Herbal supplements may contain some of the minerals that can be harmful to renal patients. There is a certain level of risk involved in the intake of these supplements without consulting a doctor and/or dietician. If you have been taking these supplements, ask your doctor if you should continue their use. Discuss it in detail with your medical care provider and ask for his approval. If they contain kidney damaging substances, then it is best to avoid them altogether. You can always take other supplements suitable for the renal diet.

Q4. What if a person has multiple medical conditions, how can he make this diet fit for all?

It is recommended to always consult a health expert and a dietician first and let them check your medical conditions. Based on the diagnosis, the dietician will create a suitable diet formula to fit all your medical conditions. Proper diagnosis is essential before adopting this renal diet.

Q5. Is it true that soaking potatoes releases their excess potassium?

There are primarily two ways to remove potassium from potatoes. Soaking the potatoes in water is one such method. The other is a double boiling method. The latter is far more effective than the former when it comes to the removal of potassium. The simple soaking does work effectively. Therefore, it is recommended to soak the potato slices into hot boiled water and leave it until it cools down, then replace it with another round of hot water, then drain to use the potatoes. The second method is to boil the potatoes in water until they turn soft. It is important to remember here that the potatoes must be peeled and diced before they are added to the boiling water. These two methods can reduce the potassium in the potatoes down to half of its original percentage. So, potato lovers are suggested to make use of these methods and enjoy potatoes as they please.

Q6. Can we use artificial sweeteners on the Renal Diet?

Yes, there are many artificial sweeteners that are not prohibited on the Renal diet. Stevia, sugar alcohols, aspartame, saccharin, and sucralose are some of the artificial sweeteners which can be freely used on the renal diet, as they do not contain any harmful additives. But it is always important to check the source and authenticity of the products you are using. It is best to consult your dietician and ask about the specific product you want to use.

Q7. How to deal with low appetite problems in CKD?

When a person suffers from renal disease, he automatically loses his appetite. It is largely because of the fluid, electrolytes, and hormonal imbalance in the body. But despite this lowering of appetite, it is important for a person to meet their caloric and protein needs to avoid malnutrition. There are a few measures you can take to overcome this problem.

> 1. Try to consume small yet frequent meals in a day. Eat something healthy after 2 or 3 hours.

2. Always take the full meal when you feel the best of your appetite. It is ok if you don't feel like eating at the exact time of lunch, dinner, or breakfast.

3. If you go out for work or some other engagements, it is best to carry some healthy snacks along with you. Eat bits of your snack every 2 hours.

4. Set an alarm or a reminder on your cellphone according to the meal and snack time and try to follow that schedule.

5. Try to add more variety to the food and add more flavors and colors to your platter. The more exciting and tempting your food will be, the better your appetite will get.

6. Do more physical activities to elevate your metabolism rate and digestion. Take a brisk walk or do some light exercise in this regard.

7. You can also ask your health expert to recommend some kidney-friendly supplements to meet the energy and protein needs of your body.

8. It does not matter how much you eat; what is important is the nutritional quality of the food you are eating. Keep that in mind every time to eat something.

CHAPTER 4:
Special Tips for a Kidney-Friendly Lifestyle

A renal diet is not a one-time magic, which makes all your renal problems go away, as it is not a one-time formula; rather, it demands constant and consistent efforts to keep your kidneys healthy. This is imperative for renal disease patients, but it is equally important for those who don't want to bear the risks of future renal damage or failure. It is therefore advised to make this diet and renal friendly lifestyle a part of your routine. It can be easily adopted by following certain important steps like the following:

- While avoiding the intake of green leafy vegetables, you should increase the intake of other kidney-friendly veggies up to about 5-9 vegetables per day.
- Replace salt with other low sodium seasonings. There are certain market products that also contain a high amount of sodium like soy sauce or readymade broths or bouillon cubes; avoid their use as well.
- Meet your protein needs by consuming more white meat and plant-based sources. It is recommended to reduce the overall protein intake to a greater extent.
- Reduce all such triggers which can cause heart diseases like saturated fats and high sugar in your diet.

- You must also avoid food which can possibly contain pesticides and environmental contaminants.
- Instead of dining out and jeopardizing your health by eating unhealthy food, it is best to eat fresh and healthy food at home.
- Avoid the use of all such additives, which may contain a high amount of sodium, potassium, and phosphorous.
- Add plenty of low sodium drinks, especially water, to your diet.
- Obesity is another major cause of kidney disease; it is important to control your weight and attain a healthy body mass index-BMI.
- Excessive use of painkillers can also damage the kidneys, so avoid using such medicines.

CHAPTER 5:
Breakfast Recipes

Onion Cheese Omelet

Cooking time: 12 minutes

Servings: 2

Ingredients:

- 3 eggs
- 1/4 cup liquid creamer
- 1 tablespoon water
- Black pepper to taste
- 1 tablespoon butter
- 3/4 cup onion, sliced
- 1 large apple, peeled, cored, and sliced
- 2 tablespoons Cheddar cheese, grated

Instructions:

- Switch your gas oven to 400 degrees F to preheat.
- Whisk the eggs with the liquid creamer, water, and black pepper in a suitable bowl.
- Stir ¼ of the butter into an oven safe skillet and sauté the onion and apple slices.
- After 5 minutes, pour in the egg mixture over the onions.

- Sprinkle Cheddar cheese over the egg and bake for approximately 12 minutes.
- Slice the omelet and serve.

Nutritional information per serving:

Calories 254

Total Fat 15.1g

Saturated Fat 7.2g

Cholesterol 268mg

Sodium 184mg

Carbohydrate 20.7g

Dietary Fiber 3.6g

Sugars 14.6g

Protein 10.9g

Calcium 98mg

Phosphorous 334mg

Potassium 280mg

Morning Patties

Cooking time: 6 minutes

Servings: 6

Ingredients:

- 1 lb. fresh lean ground chicken
- 2 teaspoons ground sage

- 2 teaspoons granulated Swerve
- 1 teaspoon ground black pepper
- ½ teaspoon ground red pepper
- 1 teaspoon basil

Instructions:

- Mix the ground chicken with the sage, Swerve, black pepper, red pepper, and basil in a suitable bowl.
- Take 2 tablespoons of this meat mixture and make a patty.
- Grease a cooking pan with cooking spray and place it over moderate heat.
- Add the patties to the pan and sear them for 2-3 minutes per side.
- Serve with fresh bread (optional).

Nutritional information per serving:

Calories 115

Total Fat 6.2g

Saturated Fat 1.8g

Cholesterol 65mg

Sodium 46mg

Carbohydrate 0.8g

Dietary Fiber 0.2g

Sugars 0.3g

Protein 13.3g

Calcium 10mg

Phosphorous 200 mg

Potassium 405mg

Maple Apple Granola

Cooking time: 50 minutes

Servings: 8

Ingredients:

- 3 jazz apples, cored and chopped
- 2 cups rolled oats
- 1 cup raw almonds, chopped
- 1/4 cup flaxseed meal
- 1 teaspoon cinnamon
- 1/3 cup butter
- 1/2 cup maple syrup
- 1 tablespoon vanilla extract

Instructions:

- Switch your gas oven to 275 degrees F to preheat.
- Take 2 large baking sheets and layer them with parchment paper.
- Mix the dry and wet ingredients separately in two bowls.
- Mix the two together to make a smooth batter.

- Divide the batter in the prepared sheets and bake them for 50 minutes.
- Slice and serve.

Nutritional information per serving:

Calories 333

Total Fat 16.2g

Saturated Fat 5.7g

Cholesterol 20mg

Sodium 60mg

Carbohydrate 42.6g

Dietary Fiber 6.7g

Sugars 21.4g

Protein 6.2g

Calcium 63mg

Phosphorous 376 mg

Potassium 325mg

Mushroom Omelet

Cooking time: 10 minutes

Servings: 2

Ingredients:

- 2 tablespoons and 1 teaspoon olive oil
- 1 shallot, minced

- ¼ lb. cremini mushrooms, rinsed
- Black pepper to taste
- 1 garlic clove, minced
- 2 teaspoons parsley, minced
- 4 eggs
- 1 tablespoon chives, minced
- 2 teaspoons milk
- 3 tablespoons Gruyere cheese, grated

Instructions:

- Set a suitable non-stick skillet over moderate heat and add 1 teaspoon olive oil.
- Add in the shallot and mushrooms, then sauté for 5 minutes until soft.
- Toss in the garlic and sauté for 1 minute.
- Now add the rest of the oil to the same skillet.
- Mix the eggs with the chives, milk, and black pepper in a bowl and pour it into the skillet.
- Cook the egg omelet for about 2 minutes per side until golden brown then transfers to the serving place.
- Serve with Gruyere cheese and parsley on top.
- Enjoy.

Nutritional information per serving:

Calories 271

Total Fat 23g

Saturated Fat 4.8g

Cholesterol 328mg

Sodium 208mg

Carbohydrate 4.8g

Dietary Fiber 0.5g

Sugars 2g

Protein 13g

Calcium 71mg

Phosphorous 227mg

Potassium 410mg

Honey Cinnamon Grapefruit

Cooking time: 6 minutes

Servings: 2

Ingredients:

- 2 teaspoons honey
- 1 grapefruit
- 1/4 teaspoon cinnamon ground

Instructions:

- Cut the grapefruit in half then slice it around its edges.
- Arrange the grapefruit in a baking tray and drizzle honey and cinnamon on top.

- Broil the grapefruit slices for 6 minutes at 400 degrees F.
- Serve warm.

Nutritional information per serving:

Calories 42

Total Fat 0.1g

Saturated Fat 0g

Cholesterol 0mg

Sodium 0mg

Carbohydrate 11.2g

Dietary Fiber 0.9g

Sugars 10.2g

Protein 0.4g

Calcium 11mg

Phosphorous 44 mg

Potassium 94mg

Chicken Egg Rolls

Cooking time: 12 minutes

Servings: 14

Ingredients:

- 1 lb. cooked chicken, diced
- 1/2 lb. bean sprouts
- 1/2 lb. cabbage, shredded

- 1 cup onion, chopped
- 2 tablespoons olive oil
- 1 tablespoon low sodium soy sauce
- 1 garlic clove, minced
- 20 egg roll wrappers
- Oil for frying

Instructions:

- Add everything to a suitable bowl except for the roll wrappers.
- Mix these ingredients well to prepare the filling then marinate for 30 minutes.
- Place the roll wrappers on the working surface and divide the prepared filling on them.
- Fold the roll wrappers as per the package instructions and keep them aside.
- Add oil to a deep wok and heat it to 350 degrees F.
- Deep the egg rolls until golden brown on all sides.
- Transfer the egg rolls to a plate lined with paper towel to absorb all the excess oil.
- Serve warm.

Nutritional information per serving:

Calories 212
Total Fat 3.8g

Saturated Fat 0.7g

Cholesterol 29mg

Sodium 329mg

Carbohydrate 29g

Dietary Fiber 1.4g

Sugars 0.9g

Protein 14.9g

Calcium 37mg

Phosphorous 361 mg

Potassium 171mg

Pork Bread Casserole

Cooking time: 55 minutes

Servings: 8

Ingredients:

- 2 tablespoons butter
- 1 lb. pork sausage
- 1 yellow onion, chopped
- 18 slices white bread, cut into cubes
- 2 ½ cups sharp Cheddar cheese, grated
- 1/2 cup fresh parsley, chopped
- 6 large eggs
- 2 cups half-and-half cream
- 1 teaspoon garlic powder

- 1/4 teaspoon black pepper

Instructions:

- Switch on your gas oven and preheat it at 325 degrees F.
- Layer a 9x9 inches casserole dish with bread cubes.
- Set a suitable-sized skillet over medium-high heat then crumb the sausage in it.
- Cook the sausage until golden brown, then keep it aside.
- Blend the eggs with the remaining ingredients in a blender until smooth.
- Stir in the sausage and spread this mixture over the bread pieces.
- Bake the bread casserole for 55 minutes approximately in the preheated oven.
- Slice and serve.
- Enjoy.

Nutritional information per serving:

Calories 366

Total Fat 26.4g

Saturated Fat 15.1g

Cholesterol 208mg

Sodium 436mg

Carbohydrate 15.2g

Dietary Fiber 0.9g

Sugars 2.1g

Protein 17.5g

Calcium 378mg

Phosphorous 501 mg

Potassium 231mg

Salmon Bagel Toast

Cooking time: 5 minutes

Servings: 2

Ingredients:

- 1 plain bagel, cut in half
- 2 tablespoons cream cheese
- 1/3 cup English cucumber, thinly sliced
- 3 oz. smoked salmon, sliced
- 3 rings red onion
- 1/2 teaspoon capers, drained

Instructions:

- Toast each half of the bagel in a skillet until golden brown.
- Cover one of the toasted halves with cream cheese.
- Set the cucumber, salmon, and capers on top of each bagel half.
- Enjoy.

Nutritional information per serving:

Calories 223

Total Fat 6.2g

Saturated Fat 2.8g

Cholesterol 21mg

Sodium 1137mg

Carbohydrate 27.5g

Dietary Fiber 1.3g

Sugars 3g

Protein 13.9g

Calcium 62mg

Phosphorous 79mg

Potassium 151mg

Cinnamon Toast Strata

Cooking time: 50 minutes

Servings: 12

Ingredients:

- 1 lb. loaf cinnamon raisin bread, cubed
- 8 oz. package cream cheese, diced
- 1 cup apples, peeled and diced
- 8 eggs
- 2 1/2 cups half-and-half cream

- 6 tablespoons butter, melted
- 1/4 cup maple syrup

Instructions:

- Layer a 9x13 inch baking dish with cooking spray.
- Place ½ of the bread cubes in the greased baking dish.
- Cover the bread cubes with cream cheese, apples, and the other half of the bread.
- Beat the eggs with the melted butter and maple syrup in a bowl.
- Pour this egg-butter mixture over the bread layer then refrigerate for 2 hours.
- Bake this bread-egg casserole for 50 minutes at 325 degrees F.
- Slice and garnish with pancake syrup.
- Enjoy.

Nutritional information per serving:

Calories 276

Total Fat 21.4g

Saturated Fat 12.4g

Cholesterol 165mg

Sodium 206mg

Carbohydrate 14.5g

Dietary Fiber 0.6g

Sugars 7.4g

Protein 7.5g

Calcium 90mg

Phosphorous 263 mg

Potassium 162mg

Cottage Cheese Pancakes

Cooking time: 10 minutes

Servings: 4

Ingredients:

- 1 cup cottage cheese
- 1/3 cup all-purpose flour
- 2 tablespoons vegetable oil
- 3 eggs, lightly beaten

Instructions:

- Begin by beating the eggs in a suitable bowl then stir in the cottage cheese.
- Once it is well mixed, stir in the flour.
- Pour a teaspoon of vegetable oil in a non-stick griddle and heat it.
- Add ¼ cup of the batter in the griddle and cook for 2 minutes per side until brown.
- Cook more of the pancakes using the remaining batter.
- Serve.

Nutritional information per serving:

Calories 196

Total Fat 11.3g

Saturated Fat 3.1g

Cholesterol 127mg

Sodium 276mg

Carbohydrate 10.3g

Dietary Fiber 0.3g

Sugars 0.5g

Protein 13g

Calcium 58mg

Phosphorous 187 mg

Potassium 110mg

Asparagus Bacon Hash

Cooking time: 27 minutes

Servings: 4

Ingredients:

- 6 slices bacon, diced
- 1/2 onion, chopped
- 2 cloves garlic, sliced
- 2 lb. asparagus, trimmed and chopped
- Black pepper, to taste

- 2 tablespoons Parmesan, grated
- 4 large eggs
- 1/4 teaspoon red pepper flakes

Instructions:

- Add the asparagus and a tablespoon of water to a microwave proof bowl.
- Cover the veggies and microwave them for 5 minutes until tender.
- Set a suitable non-stick skillet over moderate heat and layer it with cooking spray.
- Stir in the onion and sauté for 7 minutes, then toss in the garlic.
- Stir for 1 minute, then toss in the asparagus, eggs, and red pepper flakes.
- Reduce the heat to low and cover the vegetables in the pan. Top the eggs with Parmesan cheese.
- Cook for approximately 15 minutes, then slice to serve.

Nutritional information per serving:

Calories 290

Total Fat 17.9g

Saturated Fat 6.1g

Cholesterol 220mg

Sodium 256mg

Carbohydrate 11.6g

Dietary Fiber 5.1g

Sugars 5.3g

Protein 23.2g

Calcium 121mg

Phosphorous 247mg

Potassium 715mg

Cheese Spaghetti Frittata

Cooking time: 10 minutes

Servings: 6

Ingredients:

- 4 cups whole-wheat spaghetti, cooked
- 4 teaspoons olive oil
- 3 medium onions, chopped
- 4 large eggs
- ½ cup milk
- ⅓ cup Parmesan cheese, grated
- 2 tablespoons fresh parsley, chopped
- 2 tablespoons fresh basil, chopped
- ½ teaspoon black pepper
- 1 tomato, diced

Instructions:

- Set a suitable non-stick skillet over moderate heat and add in the olive oil.
- Place the spaghetti in the skillet and cook by stirring for 2 minutes on moderate heat.
- Whisk the eggs with milk, parsley, and black pepper in a bowl.
- Pour this milky egg mixture over the spaghetti and top it all with basil, cheese, and tomato.
- Cover the spaghetti frittata again with a lid and cook for approximately 8 minutes on low heat.
- Slice and serve.

Nutritional information per serving:

Calories 230
Total Fat 7.8g
Saturated Fat 2g
Cholesterol 127mg
Sodium 77mg
Carbohydrate 31.9g
Dietary Fiber 5.6g
Sugars 4.5g
Protein 11.1g
Calcium 88mg
Phosphorous 368 mg
Potassium 214mg

Pineapple Bread

Cooking time: 1 hour

Servings: 10

Ingredients:

- 1/3 cup Swerve
- 1/3 cup butter, unsalted
- 2 eggs
- 2 cups flour
- 3 teaspoons baking powder
- 1 cup pineapple, undrained
- 6 cherries, chopped

Instructions:

- Whisk the Swerve with the butter in a mixer until fluffy.
- Stir in the eggs, then beat again.
- Add the baking powder and flour, then mix well until smooth.
- Fold in the cherries and pineapple.
- Spread this cherry-pineapple batter in a 9x5 inch baking pan.
- Bake the pineapple batter for 1 hour at 350 degrees F.
- Slice the bread and serve.

Nutritional information per serving:

Calories 197

Total Fat 7.2g

Saturated Fat 1.3g

Cholesterol 33mg

Sodium 85mg

Carbohydrate 18.3g

Dietary Fiber 1.1g

Sugars 3 g

Protein 4g

Calcium 79mg

Phosphorous 316mg

Potassium 227mg

Parmesan Zucchini Frittata

Cooking time: 35 minutes

Servings: 6

Ingredients:

- 1 tablespoon olive oil
- 1 cup yellow onion, sliced
- 3 cups zucchini, chopped
- ½ cup Parmesan cheese, grated
- 8 large eggs
- ½ teaspoon black pepper
- 1/8 teaspoon paprika

- 3 tablespoons parsley, chopped

Instructions:

- Toss the zucchinis with the onion, parsley, and all other ingredients in a large bowl.
- Pour this zucchini-garlic mixture in an 11x7 inches pan and spread it evenly.
- Bake the zucchini casserole for approximately 35 minutes at 350 degrees F.
- Cut in slices and serve.

Nutritional information per serving:

Calories 142

Total Fat 9.7g

Saturated Fat 2.8g

Cholesterol 250mg

Sodium 123mg

Carbohydrate 4.7g

Dietary Fiber 1.3g

Sugars 2.4g

Protein 10.2g

Calcium 73mg

Phosphorous 375mg

Potassium 286mg

Texas Toast Casserole

Cooking time: 30 minutes

Servings: 10

Ingredients:

- 1/2 cup butter, melted
- 1 cup brown Swerve
- 1 lb. Texas Toast bread, sliced
- 4 large eggs
- 1 1/2 cup milk
- 1 tablespoon vanilla extract
- 2 tablespoons Swerve
- 2 teaspoons cinnamon
- Maple syrup for serving

Instructions:

- Layer a 9x13 inches baking pan with cooking spray.
- Spread the bread slices at the bottom of the prepared pan.
- Whisk the eggs with the remaining ingredients in a mixer.
- Pour this mixture over the bread slices evenly.
- Bake the bread for 30 minutes at 350 degrees F in a preheated oven.

- Serve.

Nutritional information per serving:

Calories 332

Total Fat 13.7g

Saturated Fat 6.9g

Cholesterol 102mg

Sodium 350mg

Carbohydrate 22.6g

Dietary Fiber 2g

Sugars 6g

Protein 7.4g

Calcium 143mg

Phosphorous 186mg

Potassium 74mg

Apple Cinnamon Rings

Cooking time: 20 minutes

Servings: 6

Ingredients:

- 4 large apples, cut in rings
- 1 cup flour
- ¼ teaspoon baking powder
- 1 teaspoon stevia

- ¼ teaspoon cinnamon
- 1 large egg, beaten
- 1 cup milk
- Vegetable oil, for frying

Cinnamon Topping:

- ⅓ cup of brown Swerve
- 2 teaspoons cinnamon

Instructions:

- Begin by mixing the flour with the baking powder, cinnamon, and stevia in a bowl.
- Whisk the egg with the milk in a bowl.
- Stir in the dry flour mixture and mix well until it makes a smooth batter.
- Pour oil into a wok to deep fry the rings and heat it up to 375 degrees F.
- First, dip the apple in the flour batter and deep fry until golden brown.
- Transfer the apple rings on a tray lined with paper towel.
- Drizzle the cinnamon and Swerve topping over the slices.
- Serve fresh in the morning.

Nutritional information per serving:

Calories 166

Total Fat 1.7g

Saturated Fat 0.5g

Cholesterol 33mg

Sodium 55mg

Carbohydrate 13.1g

Dietary Fiber 1.9g

Sugars 6.9g

Protein 4.7g

Calcium 65mg

Phosphorous 241mg

Potassium 197mg

Zucchini Bread

Cooking time: 1 hour

Servings: 16

Ingredients:

- 3 eggs
- 1 1/2 cups Swerve
- 1 cup apple sauce
- 2 cups zucchini, shredded
- 1 teaspoon vanilla
- 2 cups flour
- 1/4 teaspoon baking powder
- 1 teaspoon baking soda

- 1 teaspoon cinnamon
- 1/2 teaspoon ginger
- 1 cup unsalted nuts, chopped

Instructions:

- Thoroughly whisk the eggs with the zucchini, apple sauce, and the rest of the ingredients in a bowl.
- Once mixed evenly, spread the mixture in a loaf pan.
- Bake it for 1 hour at 375 degrees F in a preheated oven.
- Slice and serve.

Nutritional information per serving:

Calories 200

Total Fat 5.4g

Saturated Fat 0.9g

Cholesterol 31mg

Sodium 94mg

Carbohydrate 26.9g

Dietary Fiber 1.6g

Sugars 16.3g

Protein 4.4g

Calcium 20mg

Phosphorous 212mg

Potassium 137mg

Garlic Mayo Bread

Cooking time: 5 minutes

Servings: 16

Ingredients:

- 3 tablespoons vegetable oil
- 4 cloves garlic, minced
- 2 teaspoons paprika
- Dash cayenne pepper
- 1 teaspoon lemon juice
- 2 tablespoons Parmesan cheese, grated
- 3/4 cup mayonnaise
- 1 loaf (1 lb.) French bread, sliced
- 1 teaspoon Italian herbs

Instructions:

- Mix the garlic with the oil in a small bowl and leave it overnight.
- Discard the garlic from the bowl and keep the garlic-infused oil.
- Mix the garlic-oil with cayenne, paprika, lemon juice, mayonnaise, and Parmesan.
- Place the bread slices in a baking tray lined with parchment paper.

- Top these slices with the mayonnaise mixture and drizzle the Italian herbs on top.
- Broil these slices for 5 minutes until golden brown.
- Serve warm.

Nutritional information per serving:

Calories 217

Total Fat 7.9g

Saturated Fat 1.8g

Cholesterol 5mg

Sodium 423mg

Carbohydrate 30.3g

Dietary Fiber 1.3g

Sugars 2g

Protein 7g

Calcium 56mg

Phosphorous 347mg

Potassium 72mg

Strawberry Topped Waffles

Cooking time: 20 minutes

Servings: 5

Ingredients:

- 1 cup flour

- 1/4 cup Swerve
- 1 ¾ teaspoons baking powder
- 1 egg, separated
- ¾ cup milk
- ½ cup butter, melted
- ½ teaspoon vanilla extract
- Fresh strawberries, sliced

Instructions:

- Prepare and preheat your waffle pan following the instructions of the machine.
- Begin by mixing the flour with Swerve and baking soda in a bowl.
- Separate the egg yolks from the egg whites, keeping them in two separate bowls.
- Add the milk and vanilla extract to the egg yolks.
- Stir the melted butter and mix well until smooth.
- Now beat the egg whites with an electric beater until foamy and fluffy.
- Fold this fluffy composition in the egg yolk mixture.
- Mix it gently until smooth, then add in the flour mixture.
- Stir again to make a smooth mixture.
- Pour a half cup of the waffle batter in a preheated pan and cook until the waffle is done.
- Cook more waffles with the remaining batter.
- Serve fresh with strawberries on top.

Nutritional information per serving:

Calories 342

Total Fat 20.5g

Saturated Fat 12.5g

Cholesterol 88mg

Sodium 156mg

Carbohydrate 21g

Dietary Fiber 0.7g

Sugars 3.5g

Protein 4.8g

Calcium 107mg

Phosphorous 126mg

Potassium 233mg

Mixed Pepper Mushroom Omelet

Cooking time: 10 minutes

Servings: 2

Ingredients:

- 1/4 cup green onions, chopped
- 1/4 cup fresh mushrooms, sliced
- 1/4 cup green pepper, chopped
- 2 tablespoons butter, divided
- 5 eggs

- 1/4 teaspoon pepper
- 1/4 cup Cheddar cheese, shredded
- 1/4 cup Monterey Jack cheese, shredded

Instructions:

- Begin by sautéing all the vegetables with the butter in a pan until crispy.
- Whisk the eggs and black pepper until foamy and fluffy.
- Spread this egg mixture over the vegetables in the pan and cover with a lid.
- Cook for about 2 minutes, then flip the omelet with a spatula.
- Drizzle the cheese on top and cover the lid for 2 more minutes.
- Slice and serve.

Nutritional information per serving:

Calories 378

Total Fat 31.5g

Saturated Fat 16.4g

Cholesterol 467mg

Sodium 402mg

Carbohydrate 3.1g

Dietary Fiber 0.7g

Sugars 1.7g

Protein 21.6g

Calcium 280mg

Phosphorous 412mg

Potassium 262mg

CHAPTER 6:
Smoothie & Drink Recipes

Blackberry Sage Water

Cooking time: 0 minutes

Servings: 8

Ingredients:

- 15 medium fresh sage leaves
- 2 teaspoons stevia
- 1 cup boiling water
- 6 oz. fresh blackberries

Instructions:

- Add the sage leaves, stevia, blackberries, and water to a blender jug.
- Blend well, then strain and refrigerate to chill.
- Serve.

Nutritional information per serving:

Calories 24

Total Fat 0.3g

Saturated Fat 0.1g

Cholesterol 0mg

Sodium 1mg

Carbohydrate 2.9g

Dietary Fiber 1.6g

Sugars 1.9g

Protein 0.4g

Calcium 28mg

Phosphorous 13mg

Potassium 48mg

Berry Milk Smoothie

Cooking time: 0 minutes

Servings: 1

Ingredients:

- ½ cup fresh blueberries
- 1 medium cucumber, peeled and sliced
- ½ cup fresh strawberries
- ½ cup almond milk

Instructions:

- First, begin by mixing all the ingredients into a blender jug.
- Pulse it for 30 seconds until well blended.
- Serve chilled.

Nutritional information per serving:

Calories 170

Total Fat 1.8g

Saturated Fat 0.2g

Cholesterol 0mg

Sodium 50mg

Carbohydrate 24.7g

Dietary Fiber 4.7g

Sugars 12.7g

Protein 3.2g

Calcium 70mg

Phosphorous 19mg

Potassium 243mg

Apple-Cinnamon Water

Cooking time: 5 minutes

Servings: 8

Ingredients:

- ½ gallon water, filtered
- 3 apples, sliced
- 3 cinnamon sticks

Instructions:

- Add the water, apple slices, and cinnamon into a blender.
- Pour this apple mixture into a suitable pot and cook for about 5 minutes.
- Strain the apple-water and allow it to cool.
- Serve.

Nutritional information per serving:

Calories 46

Total Fat 0.2g

Saturated Fat 0g

Cholesterol 0mg

Sodium 8mg

Total Carbohydrate 12.2g

Dietary Fiber 2.5g

Sugars 8.7g

Protein 0.3g

Calcium 16mg

Phosphorous 36 mg

Potassium 96mg

Caramel Latte

Cooking time: 0 minutes

Servings: 1

Ingredients:

- 1/2 cup milk
- 1 tablespoon brown Swerve
- 1 tablespoon caramel topping
- 1 tablespoon caramel sauce
- 1/4 teaspoon vanilla extract
- 1 cup coffee

Instructions:

- Heat the milk in a 1-quart saucepan over moderate heat and add the Swerve, vanilla extract, and coffee.
- Cook this latte up to a boil then pour into the serving mug.
- Top it with caramel and sauce.
- Enjoy.

Nutritional information per serving:

Calories 217

Total Fat 4.3g

Saturated Fat 2.8g

Cholesterol 15mg

Sodium 166mg

Carbohydrate 32.8g

Dietary Fiber 0.2g

Sugars 16.4g

Protein 4.6g

Calcium 168mg

Phosphorous 41mg

Potassium 217mg

Strawberry Smoothie

Cooking time: 0 minutes

Servings: 1

Ingredients:

- 3/4 cup fresh strawberries
- 1/2 cup liquid egg whites, pasteurized
- 1/2 cup ice

Instructions:

- First, begin by putting everything into a blender jug.
- Pulse it for 30 seconds until well blended.
- Serve chilled.

Nutritional information per serving:

Calories 146

Total Fat 0.3g

Saturated Fat 0g

Cholesterol 0mg

Sodium 205mg

Carbohydrate 11.6g

Dietary Fiber 2.2g

Sugars 6.2g

Protein 14.1g

Calcium 21mg

Phosphorous 121mg

Potassium 166mg

Watermelon Mint Drink

Cooking time: 0 minutes

Servings: 2

Ingredients:

- 6 cups seedless watermelon, cubed
- The juice of 2 limes
- 1 cup of water

Instructions:

- First, begin by putting everything into a blender jug.
- Pulse it for 30 seconds until well blended.
- Serve chilled.

Nutritional information per serving:

Calories 148

Total Fat 0.6g

Saturated Fat 0.3g

Cholesterol 0mg

Sodium 11mg

Carbohydrate 38g

Dietary Fiber 2g

Sugars 28.7g

Protein 2.9g

Calcium 41mg

Phosphorous 24mg

Potassium 559mg

Beet Carrot Juice

Cooking time: 0 minutes

Servings: 2

Ingredients:

- 1 medium beet, peeled and quartered
- 1 medium apple, peeled, cored and quartered
- 1 tablespoon fresh ginger
- 3 whole carrots, rinsed and peeled
- ½ cup apple juice

Instructions:

- Pass the beet, apple, ginger, and carrot through a juicer, one after another.

- Pour the mix of the juices with the apple juice into two serving glasses and refrigerate to chill.
- Serve.

Nutritional information per serving:

Calories 155

Total Fat 0.5g

Saturated Fat 0.1g

Cholesterol 0mg

Sodium 106mg

Carbohydrate 38.3g

Dietary Fiber 6.4g

Sugars 26.2g

Protein 2.2g

Calcium 47mg

Phosphorous 56mg

Potassium 663mg

Cinnamon Egg Smoothie

Cooking time: 0 minutes

Servings: 2

Ingredients:

- 1/2 teaspoon ground cinnamon
- 1 teaspoon stevia

- 1/8 teaspoon vanilla extract
- 8 oz. egg white, pasteurized
- 3 tablespoons whipped topping

Instructions:

- Mix the stevia, egg whites, cinnamon, and vanilla in a mixer.
- Serve with whipped topping.
- Enjoy.

Nutritional information per serving:

Calories 95

Total Fat 1.2g

Saturated Fat 0.6g

Cholesterol 3mg

Sodium 120mg

Carbohydrate 3.1g

Dietary Fiber 0.3g

Sugars 0.8g

Protein 12.5g

Calcium 18mg

Phosphorous 185mg

Potassium 194mg

Pineapple Sorbet Smoothie

Cooking time: 0 minutes

Servings: 1

Ingredients:

- 3/4 cup pineapple sorbet
- 1 scoop protein powder
- 1/2 cup water
- 2 ice cubes, optional

Instructions:

- First, begin by putting everything into a blender jug.
- Pulse it for 30 seconds until well blended.
- Serve chilled.

Nutritional information per serving:

Calories 180

Total Fat 1g

Saturated Fat 0.5g

Cholesterol 40mg

Sodium 86mg

Carbohydrate 30.5g

Dietary Fiber 0g

Sugars 28g

Protein 13g

Calcium 9mg

Phosphorous 164mg

Potassium 111mg

Vanilla Fruit Smoothie

Cooking time: 0 minutes

Servings: 2

Ingredients:

- 2 oz. mango, peeled and cubed
- 2 oz. strawberries
- 2 oz. avocado flesh, cubed
- 2 oz. banana, peeled
- 2 scoops of protein powder
- 1 cup cold water
- 1 cup crushed ice

Instructions:

- First, begin by putting everything into a blender jug.
- Pulse it for 30 seconds until well blended.
- Serve chilled.

Nutritional information per serving:

Calories 228

Total Fat 7.6g

Saturated Fat 2.1g

Cholesterol 65mg

Sodium 58mg

Total Carbohydrate 19g

Dietary Fiber 3.6g

Sugars 9.8g

Protein 23.4g

Calcium 112mg

Phosphorous 216 mg

Potassium 504mg

Protein Berry Smoothie

Cooking time: 0 minutes

Servings: 2

Ingredients:

- 4 oz. water
- 1 cup frozen mixed berries
- 2 ice cubes
- 1 teaspoon blueberry essence
- 2 scoops whey protein powder

Instructions:

- First, begin by putting everything into a blender jug.
- Pulse it for 30 seconds until well blended.
- Serve chilled.

Nutritional information per serving:

Calories 248

Total Fat 11.4g

Saturated Fat 6.7g

Cholesterol 98mg

Sodium 67mg

Carbohydrate 13.3g

Dietary Fiber 2.5g

Sugars 6.1g

Protein 23.3g

Calcium 132mg

Phosphorous 152mg

Potassium 296mg

Protein Peach Smoothie

Cooking time: 0 minutes

Servings: 1

Ingredients:

- 1/2 cup ice
- 2 tablespoons egg whites, pasteurized

- 3/4 cup fresh peaches
- 1 teaspoon stevia

Instructions:

- First, begin by putting everything into a blender jug.
- Pulse it for 30 seconds until well blended.
- Serve chilled.

Nutritional information per serving:

Calories 195

Total Fat 0.3g

Saturated Fat 0g

Cholesterol 0mg

Sodium 347mg

Carbohydrate 17g

Dietary Fiber 1.7g

Sugars 14.2g

Protein 24.1g

Calcium 25mg

Phosphorous 233mg

Potassium 526mg

Cranberry Cucumber Smoothie

Cooking time: 0 minutes

Servings: 1

Ingredients:

- 1 cup frozen cranberries
- 1 medium cucumber, peeled and sliced
- 1 stalk of celery
- 1 teaspoon lime juice

Instructions:

- First, begin by putting everything into a blender jug.
- Pulse it for 30 seconds until well blended.
- Serve chilled.

Nutritional information per serving:

Calories 119

Total Fat 0.4g

Saturated Fat 0.1g

Cholesterol 0mg

Sodium 21mg

Carbohydrate 25.1g

Dietary Fiber 6g

Sugars 10g

Protein 2.3g

Calcium 79mg

Phosphorous 184mg

Potassium 325mg

Raspberry Smoothie

Cooking time: 0 minutes

Servings: 2

Ingredients:

- 1 cup frozen raspberries
- 1 medium peach, pitted, sliced
- ½ cup tofu
- 1 tablespoon honey
- 1 cup milk

Instructions:

- First, begin by putting everything into a blender jug.
- Pulse it for 30 seconds until well blended.
- Serve chilled.

Nutritional information per serving:

Calories 223

Total Fat 2.7g

Saturated Fat 0.3g

Cholesterol 0mg

Sodium 99mg

Carbohydrate 49.9g

Dietary Fiber 7.2g

Sugars 43.1g

Protein 3.6g

Calcium 176mg

Phosphorous 95mg

Potassium 426mg

Citrus Pineapple Shake

Cooking time: 0 minutes

Servings: 2

Ingredients:

- 1/2 cup pineapple juice
- 1/2 cup almond milk
- 1 cup orange sherbet
- 1/2 cup egg, pasteurized

Instructions:

- Pour the almond milk, pineapple juice, sherbet, and egg into the blender.
- Blend well for 1 minute then refrigerate to chill.
- Serve.

Nutritional information per serving:

Calories 242

Total Fat 8.2g

Saturated Fat 2.8g

Cholesterol 227mg

Sodium 155mg

Carbohydrate 33g

Dietary Fiber 1.1g

Sugars 26.2g

Protein 8.9g

Calcium 80mg

Phosphorous 121mg

Potassium 234mg

Pineapple Smoothie

Cooking time: 0 minutes

Servings: 2

Ingredients:

- 3/4 cup pineapple sherbet
- 1 scoop protein powder
- 1/2 cup water
- 2 ice cubes

Instructions:

- Add the water, pineapple sherbet, protein powder, and ice to a blender.

- Blend the pineapple smoothie for 1 minute.
- Serve.

Nutritional information per serving:

Calories 91

Total Fat 0.6g

Saturated Fat 0.2g

Cholesterol 7mg

Sodium 36mg

Carbohydrate 10.4g

Dietary Fiber 0g

Sugars 8g

Protein 11.9g

Calcium 208mg

Phosphorous 49mg

Potassium 25mg

Hazelnut Coffee

Cooking time: 0 minutes

Servings: 2

Ingredients:

- 4 cups brewed coffee
- 8 teaspoons hazelnut syrup
- 4 tablespoons almond milk

- 8 cinnamon sticks

Instructions:

- Begin by brewing the coffee in a coffee maker, then pour it into the 4 small serving cups.
- Add 1 tablespoon almond milk, 2 teaspoons hazelnut syrup, and 2 cinnamon sticks to each mug.
- Serve.

Nutritional information per serving:

Calories 65

Total Fat 4.5g

Saturated Fat 0.7g

Cholesterol 3mg

Sodium 24mg

Carbohydrate 4.4g

Dietary Fiber 1.8g

Sugars 1.7g

Protein 2.6g

Calcium 76mg

Phosphorous 73mg

Potassium 302mg

Lemon Piña Colada

Cooking time: 0 minutes

Servings: 1

Ingredients:

- 6 oz. pineapple juice
- 1 oz. lemon-lime juice
- 1 oz. protein powder
- 1/2 cup crushed ice
- 2 slices fresh pineapple

Instructions:

- Put the protein powder, pineapple juice, and ice into a blender jug.
- Pour the piña colada mixture into the serving glasses.
- Top the Piña Coladas with lemon-lime juice.
- Garnish with pineapple slices.
- Serve.

Nutritional information per serving:

Calories 227

Total Fat 2.2g

Saturated Fat 1.1g

Cholesterol 59mg

Sodium 60mg

Carbohydrate 31.3g

Dietary Fiber 1g

Sugars 22.5g

Protein 21.3g

Calcium 121mg

Phosphorous 94mg

Potassium 462mg

Blueberry Apple Blast

Cooking time: 0 minutes

Servings: 2

Ingredients:

- 1 cup frozen blueberries
- 6 tablespoons vanilla protein powder
- 8 ice cubes
- 14 oz. apple juice

Instructions:

- First, begin by putting everything into a blender jug.
- Pulse it for 30 seconds until well blended.
- Serve chilled.

Nutritional information per serving:

Calories 260

Total Fat 2.3g

Saturated Fat 1g

Cholesterol 65mg

Sodium 71mg

Carbohydrate 38.3g

Dietary Fiber 2g

Sugars 8.1g

Protein 23g

Calcium 113mg

Phosphorous 105mg

Potassium 495mg

Allspice Cider

Cooking time: 0 minutes

Servings: 8

Ingredients:

- 8 cups apple cider
- 3 cinnamon sticks
- 1/4 teaspoon whole cloves
- 1/4 teaspoon ground allspice

Instructions:

- Add the cider, cinnamon sticks, allspice, and cloves to a slow cooker.
- Cook this apple cider mixture for 1 hour on low heat.
- Strain and serve.

Nutritional information per serving:

Calories 118

Total Fat 0.3g

Saturated Fat 0.1g

Cholesterol 0mg

Sodium 8mg

Carbohydrate 29.3g

Dietary Fiber 0.4g

Sugars 27g

Protein 0.2g

Calcium 21mg

Phosphorous 124mg

Potassium 298mg

CHAPTER 7:
Snacks and Sides Recipes

Basic Meat Loaf

Cooking time: 45 minutes

Servings: 8

Ingredients:

- 1 lb. lean ground turkey
- 1 egg white
- 1 tablespoon lemon juice
- ½ cup plain breadcrumbs
- ½ teaspoon onion powder
- ½ teaspoon Italian seasoning
- ¼ teaspoon black pepper
- ½ cup chopped onions
- ½ cup diced green bell pepper
- ¼ cup of water

Instructions:

- Mix the meat with the lemon juice thoroughly in a bowl.
- Stir in the remaining seasoning, breadcrumbs, egg white, veggies, and water.
- Mix well, then spread this mixture in a loaf pan.

- Bake the crumbly meatloaf for 45 minutes at 350 degrees F.
- Slice and serve.

Nutritional information per serving:

Calories 118
Total Fat 4.6g
Saturated Fat 1.4g
Cholesterol 41mg
Sodium 98mg
Carbohydrate 6.5g
Dietary Fiber 0.5g
Sugars 1.3g
Protein 12.8g
Calcium 24mg
Phosphorous 241mg
Potassium 223mg

Cereal Munch

Cooking time: 45 minutes

Servings: 3

Ingredients:

- 3 cups cereal, salt-free
- 1 ½ cups oyster crackers, salt-free

- 2 ½ tablespoons butter, unsalted
- ½ cup pretzel twists, salt-free
- ½ tablespoon chili powder
- 1 pinch ground cumin
- ¼ teaspoon garlic powder
- 1 pinch cayenne pepper
- ¾ teaspoons lemon juice

Instructions:

- Brush a 10x15 inches pan with melted butter.
- Toss the pretzels and crackers with the remaining ingredients in the baking tray.
- Bake them for 45 minutes in the oven at 350 degrees F.
- Toss the cereal munch every 15 minutes.
- Serve.

Nutritional information per serving:

Calories 379

Total Fat 11.2g

Saturated Fat 1.8g

Cholesterol 0mg

Sodium 254mg

Carbohydrate 48.9g

Dietary Fiber 9.3g

Sugars 21.3g

Protein 8.3g

Calcium 28mg

Phosphorous 319mg

Potassium 365mg

Coconut Mandarin Salad

Cooking time: 0 minutes

Servings: 6

Ingredients:

- 20 oz. can pineapple chunks
- 11 oz. canned mandarin oranges
- 10 oz. maraschino cherries, cut in halves
- 16 oz. sour cream
- 2 cups shredded sweetened coconut

Instructions:

- Toss the pineapples with the cherries, oranges, coconut, and sour cream in a bowl.
- Serve fresh.

Nutritional information per serving:

Calories 372

Total Fat 24.9g

Saturated Fat 17.8g

Cholesterol 33mg

Sodium 49mg

Total Carbohydrate 36.2g

Dietary Fiber 4.3g

Sugars 28.8g

Protein 3.9g

Phosphorous 356mg

Potassium 464mg

Cream dipped Cucumbers

Cooking time: 0 minutes

Servings: 4

Ingredients:

- 1/2 cup sour cream
- 3 tablespoons white vinegar
- 1 teaspoon stevia
- Pepper to taste
- 4 cucumbers, peeled and sliced
- 1 small sweet onion, cut in rings

Instructions:

- Use a medium-sized serving bowl.
- Add in the cucumber, onion, and all the other ingredients.
- Mix them well and refrigerate for 2 hours.

- Toss again, serve and enjoy.

Nutritional information per serving:

Calories 127

Total Fat 6.4g

Saturated Fat 3.9g

Cholesterol 13mg

Sodium 23mg

Carbohydrate 9.2g

Dietary Fiber 1.9g

Sugars 4.2g

Protein 3.1g

Calcium 86mg

Phosphorous 172mg

Potassium 518mg

Barbecue Cups

Cooking time: 20 minutes

Servings: 10

Ingredients:

- ¾ lb. lean ground turkey
- ½ cup spicy barbecue sauce
- 2 teaspoons onion flakes
- 1 dash garlic powder

- 1 (10-oz.) package low-fat biscuits

Instructions:

- Grease a suitable pan with cooking spray and place it over moderate heat.
- Add the ground turkey and sauté it until golden brown.
- Flatten the biscuits and place them in a muffin tray.
- Press each biscuit in its muffin cup and divide the turkey in them.
- Top the turkey with barbecue sauce, garlic powder, and onion flakes.
- Bake for 12 minutes at 400 degrees F in a preheated oven.
- Serve.

Nutritional information per serving:

Calories 143

Total Fat 6.3g

Saturated Fat 1.8g

Cholesterol 25mg

Sodium 329mg

Carbohydrate 13.1g

Dietary Fiber 0.2g

Sugars 2.7g

Protein 8.6g

Calcium 21mg

Phosphorous 367mg

Potassium 164mg

Spiced Pretzels

Cooking time: 1 hour 15 minutes

Servings: 10

Ingredients:

- 1 teaspoon ground cayenne pepper
- 1 teaspoon lemon pepper
- 1 1/2 teaspoons garlic powder
- 1 oz. dry Ranch-style dressing
- 3/4 cup vegetable oil
- 15 oz. packages mini pretzels

Instructions:

- Switch the oven to 175 degrees F to preheat.
- Spread the pretzels on a cooking sheet and break them into pieces.
- Whisk the oil with the garlic powder, lemon pepper, ground cayenne pepper, and ranch dressing in a bowl.
- Pour this oil dressing over the pretzels and toss well to coat.
- Bake the pretzels for approximately 1 hour then flip them to bake for another 15 minutes.

- Serve fresh and warm.

Nutritional information per serving:

Calories 311

Total Fat 18.6g

Saturated Fat 3.2g

Cholesterol 0mg

Sodium 270mg

Carbohydrate 33.2g

Dietary Fiber 1.6g

Sugars 0g

Protein 3g

Calcium 1mg

Phosphorous 371mg

Potassium 6mg

Cauliflower with Mustard Sauce

Cooking time: 10 minutes

Servings: 4

Ingredients:

- 1 head cauliflower, separated into florets
- 1/2 cup mayonnaise
- 1/4 cup Dijon mustard
- 1 cup sharp Cheddar cheese, shredded

Instructions:

- Whisk the mayonnaise with the mustard and cheese in a bowl.
- Add the cauliflower florets in boiling water in a pot and cook until they are tender.
- Drain the cauliflower then toss its florets with the mayo mixture.
- Spread the cauliflower mixture in a baking pan.
- Broil it for 5 minutes until the cheese is melted.
- Serve fresh.

Nutritional information per serving:

Calories 255

Total Fat 19.9g

Saturated Fat 7.5g

Cholesterol 37mg

Sodium 582mg

Carbohydrate 11.7g

Dietary Fiber 2.2g

Sugars 3.8g

Protein 9.3g

Calcium 231mg

Phosphorous 97mg

Potassium 253mg

Pineapple Cabbage Coleslaw

Cooking time: 0 minutes

Servings: 12

Ingredients:

- 12 oz. (bag) broccoli coleslaw
- 12 oz. Napa cabbage, finely shredded
- 20 oz. (can) unsweetened pineapple, drained
- 1/2 cup green onions, sliced
- 1 cup mayonnaise
- 1 tablespoon seasoned rice vinegar
- 1 teaspoon coarse ground black pepper

Instructions:

- Toss the cabbage with the broccoli, and all the other ingredients in a salad bowl.
- Refrigerate this coleslaw for at least 1 hour.
- Serve.

Nutritional information per serving:

Calories 186
Total Fat 12.7g
Saturated Fat 2g
Cholesterol 5mg

Sodium 224mg

Carbohydrate 18g

Dietary Fiber 2.1g

Sugars 10.4g

Protein 2g

Calcium 42mg

Phosphorous 106mg

Potassium 139mg

Seafood Croquettes

Cooking time: 20 minutes

Servings: 8

Ingredients:

- 14.75 oz. packed salmon
- 2 egg whites
- ¼ cup chopped onion
- ½ teaspoon black pepper
- ½ cup plain breadcrumbs
- 2 tablespoons lemon juice
- ½ teaspoon ground mustard
- ¼ cup regular mayonnaise

Instructions:

- Drain the packed salmon and transfer it to a bowl.

- Stir in all the other ingredients except the oil and mix well.
- Make 8 patties out of this mixture and keep them aside.
- Add the oil to a pan and place it over medium-high heat.
- Add 4 patties at a time and sear them for 3 minutes per side.
- Cook the remaining four in the same manner until golden brown.
- Serve.

Nutritional information per serving:

Calories 282

Total Fat 12g

Saturated Fat 2.6g

Cholesterol 66mg

Sodium 202mg

Carbohydrate 7.4g

Dietary Fiber 0.4g

Sugars 1.3g

Protein 12.6g

Calcium 88mg

Phosphorous 137mg

Potassium 253mg

Sweet Rice Salad

Cooking time: 0 minutes

Servings: 6

Ingredients:

- 3 tablespoons apricot jam
- 1 tablespoon water
- 1 tablespoon lemon juice
- 7 tablespoons mayonnaise
- 6 oz. long-grain rice, cooked & rinsed
- 1 oz. onion, finely chopped
- 2 apples, chopped
- 8 cherry tomatoes

Instructions:

- Mix the rice with the apples, tomatoes, and onion in a salad bowl.
- Whisk the apricot jam and the rest of the dressing ingredients in a small bowl.
- Pour this dressing into the rice salad and mix well.
- Serve.

Nutritional information per serving:

Calories 265

Total Fat 6.4g

Saturated Fat 1g

Cholesterol 4mg

Sodium 137mg

Carbohydrate 49.2g

Dietary Fiber 4.3g

Sugars 17.8g

Protein 4g

Calcium 30mg

Phosphorous 258mg

Potassium 520mg

Herbed Shrimp Spread

Cooking time: 0 minutes

Servings: 8

Ingredients:

- 1/2 lb. shrimp, cooked, peeled and deveined
- 1/2 cup reduced-fat sour cream
- 1/2 cup light mayonnaise
- 2 scallions, coarsely chopped
- 1 teaspoon lemon zest, finely grated
- 2 teaspoons fresh lemon juice
- 1/4 cup parsley, chopped

Instructions:

- Begin by tossing the minced shrimp with the sour cream in a bowl.
- Add in the mayonnaise, scallions, lemon juice and lemon zest.
- Mix well and garnish with parsley.
- Serve the spread.

Nutritional information per serving:

Calories 118

Total Fat 8.3g

Saturated Fat 2.7g

Cholesterol 65mg

Sodium 177mg

Carbohydrate 4.6g

Dietary Fiber 0.2g

Sugars 1.1g

Protein 6.7g

Calcium 35mg

Phosphorous 203mg

Potassium 95mg

Almond Caramel Corn

Cooking time: 1 hour 5 minutes

Servings: 30

Ingredients:

- 12 cups popped popcorn
- 3 cups unblanched whole almonds
- 1 cup brown Swerve
- ½ cup butter
- ¼ cup light corn syrup
- ½ teaspoon baking soda

Instructions:

- Take a suitable roasting pan and spread the almonds and popcorn in it.
- Whisk the Swerve with the butter and corn syrup in a heavy saucepan.
- Stir-fry this corn syrup for about 5 minutes up to a boil then add in the baking soda.
- Pour this corn sauce over the popcorn and almonds in the pan.
- Bake the popcorn mixture for approximately 1 hour at 200 degrees F in the oven.
- Stir well then serve.

Nutritional information per serving:

Calories 120

Total Fat 8g

Saturated Fat 2.3g

Cholesterol 8mg

Sodium 45mg

Carbohydrate 6.5g

Dietary Fiber 1.7g

Sugars 1.1g

Protein 2.5g

Calcium 31mg

Phosphorous 23mg

Potassium 88mg

Jalapeno Tomato Salsa

Cooking time: 0 minutes

Servings: 4

Ingredients:

- 4 jalapeños, seeded and chopped
- 3 garlic cloves, peeled
- 1/2 white onion, chopped
- 2 lb. tomatoes, quartered
- Juice of 1/2 lime

Instructions:

- Add the jalapeños, garlic, onion, tomatoes, and lime juice into a blender.
- Blend this salsa mixture until it gets chunky.
- Serve fresh.

Nutritional information per serving:

Calories 32
Total Fat 0.3g
Saturated Fat 0g
Cholesterol 0mg
Sodium 638mg
Carbohydrate 5.3g
Dietary Fiber 1.6g
Sugars 3.2g
Protein 1.1g
Calcium 13mg
Phosphorous 33mg
Potassium 244mg

Blue Cheese Pear Salad

Cooking time: 0 minutes

Servings: 6

Ingredients:

- 1/2 cup sliced red onion

- 1 Bosc pear, cored and sliced
- 1/2 cup chopped candied pecans
- 1/2 cup crumbled blue cheese
- 1/4 cup maple syrup
- 1/3 cup apple cider vinegar
- 1/2 cup mayonnaise
- 2 tablespoons brown Swerve
- 1/4 teaspoon black pepper
- 1/4 cup olive oil

Instructions:

- Add all the pear salad ingredients to a salad bowl.
- Toss them well and refrigerate for 1 hour.
- Serve.

Nutritional information per serving:

Calories 229

Total Fat 13.8g

Saturated Fat 3.3g

Cholesterol 14mg

Sodium 300mg

Carbohydrate 20g

Dietary Fiber 1.8g

Sugars 13g

Protein 4.2g

Calcium 84mg

Phosphorous 54mg

Potassium 159mg

Sweet Popped Popcorn

Cooking time: 5 minutes

Servings: 4

Ingredients:

- 2 ¾ oz. popped popcorn
- 2 tablespoons butter
- 2 tablespoons corn syrup
- 2 tablespoons brown Swerve
- 1 teaspoon oil

Instructions:

- Whisk the corn syrup, brown Swerve and oil in a saucepan.
- Stir-fry the corn syrup mixture for 5 minutes then remove it from heat.
- Add the butter and mix well, then let the mixture cool.
- Toss in the popped popcorn.
- Serve.

Nutritional information per serving:

Calories 224

Total Fat 7.1g

Saturated Fat 3.9g

Cholesterol 15mg

Sodium 178mg

Carbohydrate 21g

Dietary Fiber 0.2g

Sugars 8.7g

Protein 1.2g

Calcium 8mg

Phosphorous 11mg

Potassium 38mg

Cranberry Pecan Salad

Cooking time: 0 minutes

Servings: 8

Ingredients:

- 1 (12 oz.) package fresh cranberries, chopped
- 1 teaspoon stevia
- 2 cups apples, chopped
- 1/2 cup pecans, chopped
- 1/2 cup vanilla yogurt
- 1 cup frozen whipped topping

Instructions:

- Add all the cranberry salad ingredients to a salad bowl.
- Toss them well and refrigerate for 1 hour.
- Serve.

Nutritional information per serving:

Calories 172

Total Fat 2.1g

Saturated Fat 1g

Cholesterol 5mg

Sodium 33mg

Carbohydrate 14.2g

Dietary Fiber 2.4g

Sugars 9.1g

Protein 1.2g

Calcium 35mg

Phosphorous 24mg

Potassium 147mg

Carrot Corn Bread

Cooking time: 30 minutes

Servings: 10

Ingredients:

- 1 1⁄4 cups unbleached flour
- 1 cup cornmeal
- 2 teaspoons baking powder
- 1 egg
- 1 1⁄4 cups milk
- 6 tablespoons pure maple syrup
- 1⁄4 cup olive oil
- 1⁄2 teaspoon pure vanilla extract
- 1⁄4 cup carrot, shredded

Instructions:

- Switch your gas oven to 400 degrees F to preheat.
- Now begin by mixing the flour with the cornmeal, baking powder, egg, milk, maple syrup, olive oil, and vanilla extract in a mixer.
- Mix well until it's smooth, then fold in the carrots.
- Stir well and evenly, then spread the batter in an 8-inch baking pan greased with cooking spray.
- Bake the batter for 30 minutes until golden brown.
- Slice and serve fresh.

Nutritional information per serving:

Calories 205

Total Fat 7.1g

Saturated Fat 1g

Cholesterol 19mg

Sodium 29mg

Carbohydrate 31.7g

Dietary Fiber 1.4g

Sugars 8.8g

Protein 4.2g

Calcium 94mg

Phosphorous 363mg

Potassium 210mg

Spiced Tortilla Chips

Cooking time: 8 minutes

Servings: 8

Ingredients:

- 4 (12-inch) flour tortillas, cut into wedges
- 4 tablespoons olive oil
- ½ teaspoon paprika
- ½ teaspoon rosemary seasoning
- ½ teaspoon cayenne pepper
- Parmesan cheese

Instructions:

- Begin by switching the oven to 425 degrees F to preheat.
- Grease the baking sheet with cooking spray.

- Add all the spices and cheese to a small bowl.
- Mix well and keep this mixture aside.
- Cut the tortillas into 8 wedges and coat them with the cheese mixture.
- Spread them on a baking tray and drizzle the remaining cheese mixture on top.
- Bake for about 8 minutes at 350 degrees F in a preheated oven.
- Serve fresh.

Nutritional information per serving:

Calories 87
Total Fat 7.4g
Saturated Fat 1.1g
Cholesterol 0mg
Sodium 5mg
Carbohydrate 5.5g
Dietary Fiber 0.8g
Sugars 0.1g
Protein 0.7g
Calcium 10mg
Phosphorous 79mg
Potassium 28mg

Tuna Dip

Cooking time: 0 minutes

Servings: 20

Ingredients:

- 2 (10 oz.) canned tuna chunks, drained
- 2 (8 oz.) packages cream cheese, softened
- 1 cup Ranch dressing
- ¾ cup pepper sauce
- 1 ½ cups shredded Cheddar cheese
- 1 bunch celery, cleaned and cut into 4-inch pieces
- 1 (8 oz.) box chicken-flavored crackers

Instructions:

- Add all the tuna dip ingredients to a salad bowl.
- Toss them well and refrigerate for 1 hour.
- Serve.

Nutritional information per serving:

Calories 256

Total Fat 14.6g

Saturated Fat 6.6g

Cholesterol 108mg

Sodium 461mg

Carbohydrate 1.4g

Dietary Fiber 0.1g

Sugars 0.4g

Protein 30.2g

Calcium 33mg

Phosphorous 147mg

Potassium 228mg

Chicken Bacon Wraps

Cooking time: 20 minutes

Servings: 4

Ingredients:

- 4 chicken breasts, boneless, skinless
- 8 slices bacon, hick-cut
- 1/4 cup brown Swerve
- 2 teaspoons smoked paprika
- 1/2 teaspoon garlic powder
- 1/4 teaspoon onion powder
- 1/2 teaspoon black pepper

Instructions:

- Wrap each chicken breast with 2 bacon slices and place them in a baking pan.
- Whisk the Swerve with all the spices and drizzle over the wrapped chicken.
- Spray the chicken with cooking oil.

- Bake it for 20 minutes at 350 degrees F in a preheated oven.
- Slice and serve.

Nutritional information per serving:

Calories 332

Total Fat 17.5g

Saturated Fat 5.8g

Cholesterol 92mg

Sodium 158mg

Carbohydrate 1.7g

Dietary Fiber 0.5g

Sugars 0.3g

Protein 32.4g

Calcium 17mg

Phosphorous 261mg

Potassium 522mg

CHAPTER 8:
Soup Recipes

Kidney Beans Taco Soup

Cooking time: 6 hours

Servings: 6

Ingredients:

- 1 lb. ground beef
- 1 cup onion, chopped
- 2 cans kidney beans
- 1 can corn
- 1 (15 oz.) can tomato
- 1 (15 oz.) can tomato sauce
- Black pepper, to taste
- 2 1/2 cups water

Instructions:

- Add the beef, onion, beans and the rest of the ingredients to a slow cooker.
- Cover the beans-corn mixture and cook for 6 hours on low temperature.
- Serve warm.

Nutritional information per serving:

Calories 228

Total Fat 5.3g

Saturated Fat 1.9g

Cholesterol 68mg

Sodium 261mg

Carbohydrate 17.6g

Dietary Fiber 4.8g

Sugars 3g

Protein 27.5g

Calcium 29mg

Phosphorous 341mg

Potassium 624mg

Squash Green Pea Soup

Cooking time: 50 minutes

Servings: 7

Ingredients:

- 5 cups butternut squash, peeled, seeded, and cubed
- 5 cups low-sodium chicken broth

Topping:

- 2 cups fresh green peas

- 2 tablespoons fresh lime juice
- Black pepper, to taste

Instructions:

- Begin by warming the broth and squash in the saucepan on moderate heat.
- Let it simmer for approximately 45 minutes then add the black pepper, lime juice, and green peas.
- Cook for another 5 minutes then allow it to cool.
- Puree the soup using the handheld blender until smooth.
- Serve.

Nutritional information per serving:

Calories 152

Total Fat 3.7g

Saturated Fat 0.3g

Cholesterol 0mg

Sodium 21mg

Carbohydrate 31g

Dietary Fiber 6.3g

Sugars 6.6g

Protein 4.2g

Calcium 156mg

Phosphorous 126mg

Potassium 366mg

Hominy Posole

Cooking time: 53 minutes

Servings: 6

Ingredients:

- 2 garlic cloves, peeled
- 1 cup boneless pork, diced
- 1 tablespoon cumin powder
- 1 onion, chopped
- 2 garlic cloves, chopped
- 2 tablespoons oil
- 1/2 teaspoon black pepper
- 1/2 teaspoon cayenne
- 2 tablespoons chili powder
- 1/4 teaspoon oregano
- 1 (29 oz.) can White Hominy, drained
- 5 cups pork broth
- 1 cup canned diced green chilis
- 2 jalapeños, chopped

Instructions:

- Set a suitable sized cooking pot over moderate heat and add the oil to heat.
- Toss in the pork pieces and sauté for 4 minutes.

- Stir in the garlic and onion, then stir-fry for 4 minutes until the onion is soft.
- Add the remaining ingredients then cover the pork soup.
- Cook for 45 minutes until the pork is tender.
- Serve warm.

Nutritional information per serving:

Calories 128

Total Fat 6.7g

Saturated Fat 1g

Cholesterol 0mg

Sodium 883mg

Carbohydrate 11.7g

Dietary Fiber 2.3g

Sugars 3.6g

Protein 5.3g

Calcium 35mg

Phosphorous 83mg

Potassium 286mg

Crab Corn Chowder

Cooking time: 12 minutes

Servings: 6

Ingredients:

- 6 bacon slices
- 2 celery ribs, diced
- 1 green bell pepper, diced
- 1 onion, diced
- 1 jalapeño pepper, seeded and diced
- 1 (32-oz.) container chicken broth
- 3 tablespoons flour
- 3 cups corn kernels
- 1 lb. crabmeat, drained
- 1 cup whipping cream
- 1/4 teaspoon pepper

Instructions:

- Add the bacon to a wok and sear it until golden brown, then transfer to a plate.
- Stir in the onion, celery and bell pepper, then sauté until soft.
- Add the corn, broth, crabmeat, cream, black pepper, and flour.
- Mix well and cook, stirring slowly for 10 minutes.
- Serve warm.

Nutritional information per serving:

Calories 330

Total Fat 15.5g

Saturated Fat 6.8g

Cholesterol 58mg

Sodium 105mg

Carbohydrate 33.5g

Dietary Fiber 3.6g

Sugars 9.3g

Protein 16.7g

Calcium 38mg

Phosphorous 146mg

Potassium 512mg

Chicken Green Beans Soup

Cooking time: 25 minutes

Servings: 4

Ingredients:

- 1 lb. chicken breasts, boneless, skinless, cubed
- 1 1/2 cups onion, sliced
- 1 1/2 cups celery, chopped
- 1 tablespoon olive oil
- 1 cup carrots, chopped
- 1 cup green beans, chopped
- 3 tablespoons flour
- 1 teaspoon dried oregano
- 2 teaspoons dried basil

- 1/4 teaspoon nutmeg
- 1 teaspoon thyme
- 32 oz. chicken broth
- 1/2 cup milk
- 2 cups frozen green peas
- 1/4 teaspoon black pepper

Instructions:

- Add the chicken to a skillet and sauté for 6 minutes, then remove it from the heat.
- Warm up the olive oil in a pan and stir-fry the onion for 5 minutes.
- Stir in the carrots, flour, green beans, basil, the sautéed chicken, thyme, oregano, and nutmeg.
- Sauté for approximately 3 minutes, then transfer the ingredients to a large pan.
- Add the milk and broth and cook until it boils.
- Stir in the green peas and cook for 5 minutes.
- Adjust seasoning with pepper and serve warm.

Nutritional information per serving:

Calories 277

Total Fat 9.6g

Saturated Fat 2.4g

Cholesterol 69mg

Sodium 586mg

Carbohydrate 17.3g

Dietary Fiber 4.5g

Sugars 6.4g

Protein 29.5g

Calcium 86mg

Phosphorous 284mg

Potassium 624mg

Cream of Corn Soup

Cooking time: 10 minutes

Servings: 3

Ingredients:

- 2 tablespoons butter
- 2 tablespoons flour
- 1/8 teaspoon black pepper
- 1 cup water
- 1 cup liquid non-dairy creamer
- 2 jars (4.5 oz. non-dairy creamer) strained baby corn

Instructions:

- Melt the butter in a saucepan then add the black pepper and flour.

- Stir well until smooth, then add the water and creamer.
- Mix well and cook until the soup bubbles.
- Add the baby corn and mix well.
- Serve.

Nutritional information per serving:

Calories 128

Total Fat 9.1g

Saturated Fat 1.3g

Cholesterol 0mg

Sodium 185mg

Carbohydrate 8.1g

Dietary Fiber 0.2g

Sugars 4g

Protein 0.6g

Calcium 6mg

Phosphorous 293mg

Potassium 11mg

Cabbage Beef Borscht

Cooking time: 2 hours

Servings: 12

Ingredients:

- 2 tablespoons vegetable oil

- 3 lbs. beef short ribs
- 1/2 cup dry red wine
- 8 cups low-sodium chicken broth
- 1/2 tablespoon berries
- 1/2 tablespoon whole black peppercorns
- 1/2 tablespoon coriander seeds
- 2 dill sprigs
- 2 oregano sprigs
- 2 parsley sprigs
- 2 tablespoons unsalted butter
- 3 beets (1 1/2 lbs.), peeled and diced
- 1 small rutabaga (1/2 lb.), peeled and diced
- 1 leek, diced
- 1 small onion, diced (1 cup)
- 1/2 lb. carrots, diced
- 2 celery ribs, diced
- 1/2 head savoy cabbage (1 lb.), cored and shredded
- 7 oz. chopped tomatoes, canned
- 1/2 cup dry red wine
- 2 tablespoons red wine vinegar
- Freshly ground pepper
- Sour cream
- Chopped dill
- Horseradish, grated, for serving

Instructions:

- Begin by placing the ribs in a large cooking pot and pour enough water to cover it.
- Cover the beef pot and cook it on a simmer until it is tender then shred it using a fork.
- Add the olive oil, rutabaga, carrots, shredded cabbage, and the remaining ingredients to the cooking liquid in the pot.
- Cover the cabbage soup and cook on low heat for 1 ½ hour.
- Serve warm.

Nutritional information per serving:

Calories 537

Total Fat 45.5g

Saturated Fat 19.8g

Cholesterol 90mg

Sodium 200mg

Carbohydrate 10g

Dietary Fiber 2.3g

Sugars 5.1g

Protein 18.7g

Calcium 60mg

Phosphorous 377mg

Potassium 269mg

Lemon Pepper Beef Soup

Cooking time: 35 minutes

Servings: 6

Ingredients:

- 1 lb. lean ground beef
- 1/2 cup onion, chopped
- 2 teaspoons lemon-pepper seasoning blend
- 1 cup beef broth
- 2 cups of water
- 1/3 cup white rice, uncooked
- 3 cups of frozen mixed vegetables
- 1 tablespoon sour cream
- Cooking oil

Instructions:

- Spray a saucepan with cooking oil and place it over moderate heat.
- Toss in the onion and ground beef, and sauté until brown.
- Stir in the broth and the rest of the ingredients then boil.
- Reduce the heat to a simmer then cover the soup to cook for another 30 minutes.
- Garnish with sour cream.
- Enjoy.

Nutritional information per serving:

Calories 252

Total Fat 5.6g

Saturated Fat 2.2g

Cholesterol 68mg

Sodium 213mg

Carbohydrate 21.3g

Dietary Fiber 4.3g

Sugars 3.4g

Protein 27.2g

Calcium 42mg

Phosphorous 359mg

Potassium 211mg

Cream of Crab Soup

Cooking time: 20 minutes

Servings: 4

Ingredients:

- 1 tablespoon unsalted butter
- 1/2 medium onion, chopped
- 1/2 lb. imitation crab meat, shredded
- 1/4 low-sodium chicken broth
- 1 cup coffee creamer

- 2 tablespoons cornstarch
- 1/8 teaspoon dillweed

Instructions:

- Add the butter to a cooking pot and melt it over moderate heat.
- Toss in the onion and sauté until soft, then stir in the crab meat.
- Stir-fry for 3 minutes then add the broth.
- Cook up to a boil then reduce the heat to low.
- Whisk the coffee creamer with the cornstarch in a bowl until smooth.
- Add this cornstarch slurry to the soup and cook until it thickens.
- Stir in the dillweed and mix gently.
- Serve warm.

Nutritional information per serving:

Calories 232

Total Fat 14.7g

Saturated Fat 7.8g

Cholesterol 51mg

Sodium 605mg

Carbohydrate 16.7g

Dietary Fiber 0.6g

Sugars 4.2g

Protein 8.1g

Calcium 69mg

Phosphorous 119mg

Potassium 146mg

Crab and Shrimp Gumbo

Cooking time: 25 minutes

Servings: 8

Ingredients:

- 1 cup bell pepper, chopped
- 1 1/2 cups onion, chopped
- 1 garlic clove, chopped
- 1/4 cup celery leaves, chopped
- 1 cup green onion tops
- 1/4 cup parsley, chopped
- 4 tablespoons olive oil
- 6 tablespoons flour
- 3 cups water
- 4 cups chicken broth
- 8 oz. shrimp, uncooked
- 6 oz. crab meat
- 1/4 teaspoon black pepper
- 1 teaspoon hot sauce
- 3 cups rice, cooked

Instructions:

- First, prepare the roux in a suitable pan by heating oil in it.
- Stir in the flour and sauté until it changes its color.
- Pour in 1 cup of water, then add the onion, garlic, celery leaves, and bell pepper.
- Cover the roux mixture and cook on low heat until the veggies turn soft.
- Add 2 more cups of water and the chicken broth, then mix again.
- Cook for 5 minutes then add the crab meat and shrimp.
- Cook for 10 minutes then add the parsley and green onion.
- Continue cooking for 5 minutes then garnish with black pepper and hot sauce.
- Serve warm with rice.

Nutritional information per serving:

Calories 423

Total Fat 9.2g

Saturated Fat 1.5g

Cholesterol 71mg

Sodium 612mg

Total Carbohydrate 47g

Dietary Fiber 2g

Sugars 2.2g

Protein 17.8g

Calcium 148mg

Phosphorous 207mg

Potassium 344mg

Beef & Vegetable Soup

Cooking time: 55 minutes

Servings: 4

Ingredients:

- 1 lb. beef stew
- 3 ½ cups water
- 1 cup raw sliced onions
- ½ cup frozen green peas
- 1 teaspoon black pepper
- ½ cup frozen okra
- ½ teaspoon basil
- ½ cup frozen carrots, diced
- ½ teaspoon thyme
- ½ cup frozen corn

Instructions:

- Place a large pot over moderate heat and add the beef, water, thyme, basil and black pepper.
- Cook the beef for 45 minutes on a simmer.
- Stir in the okra and other vegetables and cook until the meat is al dente.
- Serve warm.

Nutritional information per serving:

Calories 163
Total Fat 6.5g
Saturated Fat 2.6g
Cholesterol 18mg
Sodium 484mg
Carbohydrate 19.3g
Dietary Fiber 4.7g
Sugars 4.8g
Protein 8g
Calcium 51mg
Phosphorous 221mg
Potassium 427mg

Chicken Noodle Soup

Cooking time: 45 minutes

Servings: 6

Ingredients:

- 1 lb. chicken, cut into parts
- 1 teaspoon red pepper
- ¼ cup lemon juice
- 1 teaspoon caraway seed
- 3 ½ cups water
- 1 teaspoon oregano
- 1 tablespoon poultry seasoning
- 1/8 teaspoon stevia
- 1 teaspoon garlic powder
- ½ cup celery
- 1 teaspoon onion powder
- ½ cup green pepper
- 2 tablespoons vegetable oil
- 1 cup egg noodles
- 1 teaspoon black pepper

Instructions:

- First, rub the chicken with lemon juice and place it in a large pot.
- Add water, vegetable oil, all the spices, herbs, and the red pepper.
- Cover the chicken soup and cook for about 30 minutes.
- Stir in the noodles along with the other ingredients and cook for 15 minutes.

- Serve.

Nutritional information per serving:

Calories 213

Total Fat 7.7g

Saturated Fat 1.8g

Cholesterol 66mg

Sodium 63mg

Carbohydrate 10g

Dietary Fiber 1.4g

Sugars 1.2g

Protein 23.9g

Calcium 40mg

Phosphorous 152mg

Potassium 265mg

Serrano Yucatan Soup

Cooking time: 20 minutes

Servings: 7

Ingredients:

- 2 tablespoons olive oil
- 1 onion, chopped
- 2 garlic cloves, minced
- 1 small Serrano pepper, diced

- 7 cups chicken broth
- 14 oz. can dice tomatoes, not drained
- 4 oz. can dice green chilies, not drained
- 1/3 cup lime juice
- 14 oz. can black beans, drained and rinsed
- 1 cup frozen corn
- 2 cups cooked rice
- 2 lbs. chicken, cooked
- 1/4 cup chopped cilantro
- 1 teaspoon ground cumin
- 1 teaspoon dried bay leaf
- 1 teaspoon dried thyme
- 1/4 teaspoon cayenne pepper
- Corn tortillas (optional)

Instructions:

- Spread the corn tortillas on a baking sheet and bake them for 3 minutes at 400 degrees F.
- Set a suitably sized saucepan over moderate heat and add the oil to heat.
- Toss in the chili peppers, garlic, and onion, then sauté until soft.
- Stir in the broth, tomatoes, beans, corn, bay leaf, and chicken.
- Let the chicken soup cook for 10 minutes on a simmer.

- Stir in the cilantro and all other ingredients.
- Cook the Serrano soup for another 1 minute.
- Garnish with baked corn tortillas.
- Serve.

Nutritional information per serving:

Calories 382

Total Fat 7.1g

Saturated Fat 1.5g

Cholesterol 70mg

Sodium 765mg

Total Carbohydrate 42.1g

Dietary Fiber 3.2g

Sugars 2.2g

Protein 35.3g

Calcium 55mg

Phosphorous 247mg

Potassumi 571mg

Mushroom Vegetable Soup

Cooking time: 50 minutes

Servings: 4

Ingredients:

- 1 cup green beans, chopped

- 3/4 cup celery, chopped
- 1/2 cup onion, chopped
- 1/2 cup carrots, chopped
- 1/2 cup mushrooms, chopped
- 1/2 cup frozen corn
- 1 medium Roma tomato, chopped
- 2 tablespoons olive oil
- 1/2 cup frozen corn
- 4 cups vegetable broth
- 1 teaspoon dried oregano leaves
- 1 teaspoon garlic powder

Instructions:

- Set a suitable cooking pot over moderate heat and add the olive oil to heat.
- Toss in the onion and celery, then sauté until soft.
- Stir in the corn and the rest of the ingredients and cook the soup up to a boil.
- Now reduce the heat to a simmer and cook for 45 minutes.
- Serve warm.

Nutritional information per serving:

Calories 147

Total Fat 8.8g

Saturated Fat 1.5g

Cholesterol 0mg

Sodium 795mg

Carbohydrate 11.5g

Dietary Fiber 2.9g

Sugars 4g

Protein 7g

Calcium 42mg

Phosphorous 297mg

Potassium 506mg

Ivory Fish Soup

Cooking time: 55 minutes

Servings: 4

Ingredients:

- 2 medium fresh white fish fillets
- 2 medium eggplants, diced
- 1 small onion, finely chopped
- 5 cloves garlic, crushed
- 1 tablespoon tomato puree
- 1 hot chili pepper

Instructions:

- Add the water and the eggplants in a large pan and cook up to a boil.
- After 10 minutes of boiling, drain the eggplants and transfer them to a pot.
- Add everything else to this pot and add enough water to cover them.
- Cook the soup on a simmer for 45 minutes.
- Serve warm.

Nutritional information per serving:

Calories 236

Total Fat 9.3g

Saturated Fat 0.9g

Cholesterol 59mg

Sodium 52mg

Carbohydrate 12.9g

Dietary Fiber 2.4g

Sugars 1g

Protein 23.1g

Calcium 37mg

Phosphorous 309mg

Potassium 370mg

Jamaican Soup

Cooking time: 1 hour

Servings: 4

Ingredients:

- 1 lb. chicken pieces
- 3 spring onions, peeled and sliced
- 4 oz. pumpkin, peeled and cut into chunks
- ½ clove garlic, chopped
- ½ cup potato, peeled and cut into chunks
- 1 medium carrot, peeled and sliced
- 1 (5 oz.) yellow yam, peeled and diced
- ½ sprig fresh thyme
- 1 teaspoon chili powder
- ½ reduced-salt chicken stock cube

For the dumplings:

- 4 oz. plain flour
- 1/4 cup cold water

Instructions:

- Mix the flour with enough water to make a smooth dumpling dough.
- Knead the dough well and divide it into golf-ball-sized pieces.
- Roll the balls in your palms first, then flatten them into a dumpling.

- Add the chicken, garlic, and pumpkin to a cooking pot and pour enough water to cover them.
- Cook this soup up to a boil, then cover and let it simmer for 15 minutes.
- Remove the lid, add the remaining veggies and continue cooking for 15 minutes.
- Stir in the dumplings and the rest of the ingredients. Cook for 30 minutes.
- Serve warm.

Nutritional information per serving:

Calories 442

Total Fat 9.3g

Saturated Fat 2.6g

Cholesterol 101mg

Sodium 151mg

Carbohydrate 43.8g

Dietary Fiber 5.8g

Sugars 2.6g

Protein 37.9g

Calcium 61mg

Phosphorous 107mg

Potassium 346mg

Cucumber Onion Soup

Cooking time: 0 minutes

Servings: 4

Ingredients:

- 2 medium cucumbers, peeled and diced
- 1/3 cup sweet white onion, diced
- 1 green onion, diced
- 2 tablespoons fresh dill
- 2 tablespoons lemon juice
- 2/3 cup water
- 1/2 cup half and half cream,
- 1/3 cup sour cream
- 1/2 teaspoon pepper

Instructions:

- Begin by tossing all the ingredients into a food processor.
- Puree the mixture and refrigerate for 2 hours.
- Garnish with dill sprigs.
- Enjoy fresh.

Nutritional information per serving:

Calories 114
Total Fat 7.8g
Saturated Fat 4.8g
Cholesterol 20mg
Sodium 33mg

Carbohydrate 10g

Dietary Fiber 1.4g

Sugars 3.3g

Protein 3.1g

Calcium 113mg

Phosphorous 240mg

Potassium 377mg

Potato Carrot Soup

Cooking time: 6 hours

Servings: 4

Ingredients:

- 1 leek
- ¾ cup potatoes, diced and boiled
- ¾ cup carrots, diced and boiled
- 1 garlic clove
- 1 tablespoon oil
- Black pepper to taste
- 3 cups low sodium chicken stock
- 1 bay leaf
- ¼ teaspoon ground cumin

Instructions:

- Add all the veggies, stock, oil, black pepper, cumin, and bay leaf to a slow cooker.
- Put the lid on and cook for 6 hours on low heat.
- Discard the bay leaf then puree the soup until smooth.
- Serve warm.

Nutritional information per serving:

Calories 85

Total Fat 3.5g

Saturated Fat 0.5g

Cholesterol 0mg

Sodium 73mg

Carbohydrate 10.8g

Dietary Fiber 1.7g

Sugars 2.2g

Protein 2.5g

Calcium 26mg

Phosphorous 172mg

Potassium 227mg

Sockeye Salmon Soup

Cooking time: 20 minutes

Servings: 4

Ingredients:

- 2 tablespoons unsalted butter, melted
- 1 medium carrot, diced
- 1/2 cup celery, chopped
- 1/2 cup onion, sliced
- 1 lb. sockeye salmon, cooked, diced
- 2 cups reduced-sodium chicken broth
- 2 cups milk
- 1/8 teaspoon black pepper
- 1/4 cup arrowroot powder
- 1/4 cup water

Instructions:

- Add the melted butter to a saucepan and sauté all the vegetables in it until soft.
- Stir in the salmon chunks, milk, black pepper, and broth.
- First cook up to boil then cook on low heat.
- Mix the arrowroot powder with water and add this slurry to the soup.
- Cook by stirring until it thickens.
- Serve fresh and warm.

Nutritional information per serving:

Calories 321

Total Fat 14.7g

Saturated Fat 5.6g

Cholesterol 71mg

Sodium 548mg

Carbohydrate 15.8g

Dietary Fiber 0.9g

Sugars 8.2g

Protein 29g

Calcium 206mg

Phosphorous 148mg

Potassium 327mg

Roasted Pepper Soup

Cooking time: 35 minutes

Servings: 4

Ingredients:

- 4 cups low-sodium chicken broth
- 3 red peppers, roasted and sliced
- 2 onions, halved and sliced
- 3 tablespoons lemon juice
- 1 tablespoon lemon zest
- 1 pinch cayenne pepper
- ¼ teaspoon cinnamon

Instructions:

- Start by putting all the soup ingredients in a saucepan.

- Cook up to a boil then reduce the heat to a simmer.
- Continue to cook on a simmer for 30 minutes.
- Serve warm.

Nutritional information per serving:

Calories 110

Total Fat 0.7g

Saturated Fat 0.2g

Cholesterol 0mg

Sodium 157mg

Carbohydrate 19.8g

Dietary Fiber 3.9g

Sugars 8.9g

Protein 6.8g

Calcium 44mg

Phosphorous 269mg

Potassium 440mg

CHAPTER 9:
Salad Recipes

Italian Cucumber Salad

Cooking time: 0 minutes

Servings: 2

Ingredients:

- 1/4 cup rice vinegar
- 1/8 teaspoon stevia
- 1/2 teaspoon olive oil
- 1/8 teaspoon black pepper
- 1/2 cucumber, sliced
- 1 cup carrots, sliced
- 2 tablespoons green onion, sliced
- 2 tablespoons red bell pepper, sliced
- 1/2 teaspoon Italian seasoning blend

Instructions:

- Put all the salad ingredients into a suitable salad bowl.
- Toss them well and refrigerate for 1 hour.
- Serve.

Nutritional information per serving:

Calories 112

Total Fat 1.6g

Saturated Fat 0.2g

Cholesterol 0mg

Sodium 43mg

Carbohydrate 8.2g

Dietary Fiber 3.5g

Sugars 4.8g

Protein 2.3g

Calcium 45mg

Phosphorous 198mg

Potassium 529mg

Grapes Jicama Salad

Cooking time: 0 minutes

Servings: 2

Ingredients:

- 1 jicama, peeled and sliced
- 1 carrot, sliced
- 1/2 medium red onion, sliced
- 1 ¼ cup seedless grapes
- 1/3 cup fresh basil leaves
- 1 tablespoon apple cider vinegar
- 1 ½ tablespoon lemon juice

- 1 ½ tablespoon lime juice

Instructions:

- Put all the salad ingredients into a suitable salad bowl.
- Toss them well and refrigerate for 1 hour.
- Serve.

Nutritional information per serving:

Calories 203

Total Fat 0.7g

Saturated Fat 0.2g

Cholesterol 0mg

Sodium 44mg

Carbohydrate 48.2g

Dietary Fiber 18.4g

Sugars 19.1g

Protein 3.7g

Calcium 79mg

Phosphorous 141mg

Potassium 429mg

Cucumber Couscous Salad

Cooking time: 0 minutes

Servings: 4

Ingredients:

- 1 cucumber, sliced
- ½ cup red bell pepper, sliced
- ¼ cup sweet onion, sliced
- 2 tablespoons black olives, sliced
- ¼ cup parsley, chopped
- ½ cup couscous, cooked
- 2 tablespoons olive oil
- 2 tablespoons rice vinegar
- 2 tablespoons feta cheese crumbled
- 1 ½ teaspoon dried basil
- 1/4 teaspoon black pepper

Instructions:

- Put all the salad ingredients into a suitable salad bowl.
- Toss them well and refrigerate for 1 hour.
- Serve.

Nutritional information per serving:

Calories 202

Total Fat 9.8g

Saturated Fat 2.4g

Cholesterol 5mg

Sodium 258mg

Carbohydrate 22.4g

Dietary Fiber 2.1g

Sugars 2.3g

Protein 6.2g

Calcium 80mg

Phosphorous 192mg

Potassium 209mg

Carrot Jicama Salad

Cooking time: 0 minutes

Servings: 2

Ingredients:

- 2 cup carrots, julienned
- 1 1/2 cups jicama, julienned
- 2 tablespoons lime juice
- 1 tablespoon olive oil
- ½ tablespoon apple cider
- ½ teaspoon brown Swerve

Instructions:

- Put all the salad ingredients into a suitable salad bowl.
- Toss them well and refrigerate for 1 hour.
- Serve.

Nutritional information per serving:

Calories 173

Total Fat 7.1g

Saturated Fat 0.5g

Cholesterol 0mg

Sodium 80mg

Carbohydrate 20.7g

Dietary Fiber 5.9g

Sugars 7.7g

Protein 1.6g

Calcium 50mg

Phosphorous 96mg

Potassium 501mg

Butterscotch Apple Salad

Cooking time: 0 minutes

Servings: 6

Ingredients:

- 3 cups jazz apples, chopped
- 8 oz. canned crushed pineapple
- 8 oz. whipped topping
- 1/2 cup butterscotch topping
- 1/3 cup almonds
- 1/4 cup butterscotch chips

Instructions:

- Put all the salad ingredients into a suitable salad bowl.
- Toss them well and refrigerate for 1 hour.
- Serve.

Nutritional information per serving:

Calories 293

Total Fat 12.7g

Saturated Fat 5.8g

Cholesterol 29mg

Sodium 152mg

Carbohydrate 45.5g

Dietary Fiber 4.2g

Sugars 19.6g

Protein 4.2g

Calcium 65mg

Phosphorous 202mg

Potassium 296mg

Cranberry Cabbage Slaw

Cooking time: 0 minutes

Servings: 4

Ingredients:

- 1/2 medium cabbage head, shredded
- 1 medium red apple, shredded
- 2 tablespoons onion, sliced
- 1/2 cup dried cranberries
- 1/4 cup almonds, toasted sliced
- 1/2 cup olive oil
- ¼ teaspoon stevia
- 1/4 cup cider vinegar
- 1/2 tablespoon celery seed
- 1/2 teaspoon dry mustard
- ½ cup cream

Instructions:

- Take a suitable salad bowl.
- Start tossing in all the ingredients.
- Mix well and serve.

Nutritional information per serving:

Calories 308

Total Fat 24.5g

Saturated Fat 4g

Cholesterol 8mg

Sodium 23mg

Carbohydrate 13.5g

Dietary Fiber 3.2g

Sugars 7.3g

Protein 2.6g

Calcium 69mg

Phosphorous 257mg

Potassium 219mg

Chestnut Noodle Salad

Cooking time: 0 minutes

Servings: 6

Ingredients:

- 8 cups cabbage, shredded
- 1/2 cup canned chestnuts, sliced
- 6 green onions, chopped
- 1/4 cup olive oil
- 1/4 cup apple cider vinegar
- 3/4 teaspoon stevia
- 1/8 teaspoon black pepper
- 1 cup chow Mein noodles, cooked

Instructions:

- Take a suitable salad bowl.
- Start tossing in all the ingredients.
- Mix well and serve.

Nutritional information per serving:

Calories 191

Total Fat 13g

Saturated Fat 1.3g

Cholesterol 1mg

Sodium 78mg

Carbohydrate 5.8g

Dietary Fiber 3.4g

Sugars 2.6g

Protein 4.2g

Calcium 142mg

Phosphorous 188mg

Potassium 302mg

Cranberry Broccoli Salad

Cooking time: 0 minutes

Servings: 4

Ingredients:

- 3/4 cup plain Greek yogurt
- 1/4 cup mayonnaise
- 2 tablespoons maple syrup
- 2 tablespoons apple cider vinegar
- 4 cups broccoli florets

- 1 medium apple, chopped
- 1/2 cup red onion, sliced
- 1/4 cup parsley, chopped
- 1/2 cup dried cranberries
- 1/4 cup pecans

Instructions:

- Put all the salad ingredients into a suitable salad bowl.
- Toss them well and refrigerate for 1 hour.
- Serve.

Nutritional information per serving:

Calories 252

Total Fat 10.5g

Saturated Fat 1.4g

Cholesterol 8mg

Sodium 157mg

Carbohydrate 34g

Dietary Fiber 5g

Sugars 22.4g

Protein 9.4g

Calcium 106mg

Phosphorous 291mg

Potassium 480mg

Balsamic Beet Salad

Cooking time: 0 minutes

Servings: 2

Ingredients:

- 1 cucumber, peeled and sliced
- 15 oz. canned low-sodium beets, sliced
- 4 teaspoon balsamic vinegar
- 2 teaspoon sesame oil
- 2 tablespoons Gorgonzola cheese

Instructions:

- Take a suitable salad bowl.
- Start tossing in all the ingredients.
- Mix well and serve.

Nutritional information per serving:

Calories 145
Total Fat 7.8g
Saturated Fat 2.4g
Cholesterol 10mg
Sodium 426mg
Carbohydrate 16.4g
Dietary Fiber 3.8g

Sugars 11.1g

Protein 5g

Calcium 109mg

Phosphorous 79mg

Potassium 229mg

Shrimp Salad

Cooking time: 0 minutes

Servings: 4

Ingredients:

- 1 lb. shrimp, boiled and chopped
- 1 hardboiled egg, chopped
- 1 tablespoon celery, chopped
- 1 tablespoon green pepper, chopped
- 1 tablespoon onion, chopped
- 2 tablespoons mayonnaise
- 1 teaspoon lemon juice
- ½ teaspoon chili powder
- ⅛ teaspoon hot sauce
- ½ teaspoon dry mustard
- Lettuce, chopped or shredded

Instructions:

- Take a suitable salad bowl.

- Start tossing in all the ingredients.
- Mix well and serve.

Nutritional information per serving:

Calories 184

Total Fat 5.7g

Saturated Fat 1.3g

Cholesterol 282mg

Sodium 381mg

Carbohydrate 4.3g

Dietary Fiber 0.3g

Sugars 0.8g

Protein 27.5g

Vitamin D 4mcg

Calcium 114mg

Phosphorous 249mg

Potassium 233mg

Chicken Cranberry Sauce Salad

Cooking time: 0 minutes

Servings: 6

Ingredients:

- 3 cups of chicken meat, cooked, cubed
- 1 cup grapes

- 2 cups carrots, shredded
- 1/4 red onion, chopped
- 1 large yellow bell pepper, chopped
- 1/4 cup mayonnaise
- 1/2 cup cranberry sauce

Instructions:

- Put all the salad ingredients into a suitable salad bowl.
- Toss them well and refrigerate for 1 hour.
- Serve.

Nutritional information per serving:

Calories 240

Total Fat 8.6g

Saturated Fat 1.9g

Cholesterol 65mg

Sodium 161mg

Carbohydrate 19.4g

Dietary Fiber 1.4g

Sugars 12.8g

Protein 21g

Calcium 31mg

Phosphorous 260mg

Potassium 351mg

Egg Celery Salad

Cooking time: 0 minutes

Servings: 4

Ingredients:

- 4 eggs, boiled, peeled and chopped
- 1/4 cup celery, chopped
- 1/2 cup sweet onion, chopped
- 2 tablespoons sweet pickle, chopped
- 3 tablespoons mayonnaise
- 1 tablespoon mustard

Instructions:

- Put all the salad ingredients into a suitable salad bowl.
- Toss them well and refrigerate for 1 hour.
- Serve.

Nutritional information per serving:

Calories 134

Total Fat 8.9g

Saturated Fat 2.1g

Cholesterol 189mg

Sodium 259mg

Carbohydrate 7.4g

Dietary Fiber 0.6g

Sugars 4g

Protein 6.8g

Calcium 36mg

Phosphorous 357mg

Potassium 113mg

Chicken Orange Salad

Cooking time: 0 minutes

Servings: 4

Ingredients:

- 1 ½ cup chicken, cooked and diced
- ½ cup celery, diced
- ½ cup green pepper, chopped
- ¼ cup onion, sliced
- 1 cup orange, peeled and cut into segments
- ¼ cup mayonnaise
- ½ teaspoon black pepper

Instructions:

- Take a suitable salad bowl.
- Start tossing in all the ingredients.
- Mix well and serve.

Nutritional information per serving:

Calories 167

Total Fat 6.6g

Saturated Fat 1.2g

Cholesterol 44mg

Sodium 151mg

Carbohydrate 11.2g

Dietary Fiber 1.1g

Sugars 7.2g

Protein 16g

Calcium 25mg

Phosphorous 211mg

Potassium 249mg

Almond Pasta Salad

Cooking time: 0 minutes

Servings: 14

Ingredients:

- 1 lb. elbow macaroni, cooked
- 1/2 cup sun-dried tomatoes, diced
- 1 (15 oz.) can whole artichokes, diced
- 1 orange bell pepper, diced
- 3 green onions, sliced

- 2 tablespoons basil, sliced
- 2 oz. slivered almonds

Dressing:

- 1 garlic clove, minced
- 1 tablespoon Dijon mustard
- 1 tablespoon raw honey
- 1/4 cup white balsamic vinegar
- 1/3 cup olive oil

Instructions:

- Take a suitable salad bowl.
- Start tossing in all the ingredients.
- Mix well and serve.

Nutritional information per serving:

Calories 260

Total Fat 7.7g

Saturated Fat 0.8g

Cholesterol 0mg

Sodium 143mg

Carbohydrate 41.4g

Dietary Fiber 9.5g

Sugars 5.2g

Protein 9.6g

Calcium 44mg

Phosphorous 39mg

Potassium 585mg

Pineapple Berry Salad

Cooking time: 0 minutes

Servings: 4

Ingredients:

- 4 cups pineapple, peeled and cubed
- 3 cups strawberries, chopped
- 1/4 cup honey
- 1/2 cup basil leaves
- 1 tablespoon lemon zest
- 1/2 cup blueberries

Instructions:

- Take a suitable salad bowl.
- Start tossing in all the ingredients.
- Mix well and serve.

Nutritional information per serving:

Calories 128

Total Fat 0.6g

Saturated Fat 0g

Cholesterol 0mg

Sodium 3mg

Carbohydrate 33.1g

Dietary Fiber 5.2g

Sugars 23.4g

Protein 1.8g

Calcium 40mg

Phosphorous 151mg

Potassium 362mg

Green & Yellow Bean Salad

Cooking time: 0 minutes

Servings: 4

Ingredients:

- 1 cup green beans, fresh
- 1 cup yellow beans, fresh
- 1/3 cup onion, sliced
- 1/3 cup green pepper, sliced
- ¼ cup olive oil
- ¼ cup vinegar
- ½ teaspoon basil, dried
- 1 teaspoon parsley, dried
- ¼ teaspoon black pepper

Instructions:

- Take a suitable salad bowl.
- Start tossing in all the ingredients.
- Mix well and serve.

Nutritional information per serving:

Calories 189

Total Fat 13.1g

Saturated Fat 1.9g

Cholesterol 0mg

Sodium 5mg

Carbohydrate 14.6g

Dietary Fiber 5.9g

Sugars 1g

Protein 4.8g

Calcium 43mg

Phosphorous 147mg

Potassium 243mg

Carrot Zucchini Salad

Cooking time: 0 minutes

Servings: 2

Ingredients:

- 1/4 cup unseasoned rice vinegar
- 1/8 teaspoon stevia
- 1/2 teaspoon olive oil
- 1/8 teaspoon black pepper
- 1/2 zucchini, peeled and julienned
- 1 cup carrots, julienned
- 2 tablespoons red bell pepper, julienned

Instructions:

- Take a suitable salad bowl.
- Start tossing in all the ingredients.
- Mix well and serve.

Nutritional information per serving:

Calories 92

Total Fat 1.6g

Saturated Fat 0.2g

Cholesterol 0mg

Sodium 43mg

Carbohydrate 6.1g

Dietary Fiber 3.5g

Sugars 3.7g

Protein 2.3g

Calcium 45mg

Phosphorous 147mg

Potassium 529mg

Broccoli Lettuce Salad

Cooking time: 0 minutes

Servings: 2

Ingredients:

- 1 cup lettuce, chopped
- ¼ zucchini, peeled and cubed
- 4 carrots, diced
- 1/4 cup broccoli florets
- 2 tablespoons balsamic vinegar
- 1 teaspoon olive oil

Instructions:

- Take a suitable salad bowl.
- Start tossing in all the ingredients.
- Mix well and serve.

Nutritional information per serving:

Calories 43
Total Fat 2.5g
Saturated Fat 0.3g
Cholesterol 0mg
Sodium 22mg
Carbohydrate 4.8g

Dietary Fiber 1.2g

Sugars 2.1g

Protein 0.8g

Calcium 19mg

Phosphorous 200mg

Potassium 188mg

Pepper Cabbage Slaw

Cooking time: 0 minutes

Servings: 4

Ingredients:

- 1 small cabbage head, shredded
- 1 medium green bell pepper, shredded
- 2 medium carrots, shredded
- 1/3 tablespoon stevia
- 1/2 cup vinegar
- 1/2 cup water
- 2 teaspoons celery seed

Instructions:

- Take a suitable salad bowl.
- Start tossing in all the ingredients.
- Mix well and serve.

Nutritional information per serving:

Calories 168

Total Fat 0.5g

Saturated Fat 0.1g

Cholesterol 0mg

Sodium 58mg

Carbohydrate 27.9g

Dietary Fiber 5.7g

Sugars 19.6g

Protein 3g

Calcium 105mg

Phosphorous 133mg

Potassium 493mg

Summer Potato Salad

Cooking time: 0 minutes

Servings: 4

Ingredients:

- 2 ¼ cups potato, boiled, peeled and diced
- 3 tablespoons celery, chopped
- 3 tablespoons onion, chopped
- 3 tablespoons green pepper, chopped
- 2 chopped hard-boiled eggs, peeled and diced

- ¼ cup mayonnaise
- 2 teaspoons vinegar
- 1⁄8 teaspoon dry mustard
- 1⁄8 teaspoon dried parsley
- 1⁄8 teaspoon paprika
- 1 pinch pepper
- 1 pinch garlic powder

Instructions:

- Take a suitable salad bowl.
- Start tossing in all the ingredients.
- Mix well and serve.

Nutritional information per serving:

Calories 128

Total Fat 7.2g

Saturated Fat 1.4g

Cholesterol 86mg

Sodium 143mg

Carbohydrate 12.4g

Dietary Fiber 1.4g

Sugars 2.1g

Protein 4g

Calcium 25mg

Phosphorous 192mg

Potassium 252mg

CHAPTER 10:
Seafood Recipes

Saucy Dill Fish

Cooking time: 15 minutes

Servings: 4

Ingredients:

- 4 (4 oz.) salmon fillets

Dill Sauce:

- 1 cup whipped cream cheese
- 4 minced garlic cloves
- ½ small onion, diced
- 3 tablespoons fresh or dried dill (as desired)
- ½ teaspoon ground pepper
- 1 teaspoon Mrs. Dash (optional)
- 2 drops of hot sauce (optional)

Instructions:

- Place the salmon fillets in a moderately shallow baking stray.

- Whisk the cream cheese and all the dill-sauce ingredients in a bowl.
- Spread the dill-sauce over the fillets liberally.
- Cover the fillet pan with a foil sheet and bake for 15 minutes at 350 degrees F.
- Serve warm.

Nutritional information per serving:

Calories 432

Total Fat 26.7g

Saturated Fat 12.9g

Cholesterol 142mg

Sodium 280mg

Carbohydrate 5g

Dietary Fiber 0.9g

Sugars 2.25g

Protein 35.8g

Calcium 141mg

Phosphorous 265mg

Potassium 590mg

Lemon Pepper Trout

Cooking time: 15 minutes

Servings: 2

Ingredients:

- 1 lb. trout fillets
- 1 lb. asparagus
- 3 tablespoons olive oil
- 5 garlic cloves, minced
- 1/2 teaspoon black pepper
- 1/2 lemon, sliced

Instructions:

- Prepare and preheat the gas oven at 350 degrees F.
- Rub the washed and dried fillets with oil then place them in a baking tray.
- Top the fish with lemon slices, black pepper, and garlic cloves.
- Spread the asparagus around the fish.
- Bake the fish for 15 minutes approximately in the preheated oven.
- Serve warm.

Nutritional information per serving:

Calories 336

Total Fat 20.3g

Saturated Fat 3.2g

Cholesterol 84mg

Sodium 370mg

Carbohydrate 6.5g

Dietary Fiber 2.7g

Sugars 2.4g

Protein 33g

Calcium 100mg

Phosphorous 107mg

Potassium 383mg

Salmon Stuffed Pasta

Cooking time: 35 minutes

Servings: 24

Ingredients:

- 24 jumbo pasta shells, boiled
- 1 cup coffee creamer

Filling:

- 2 eggs, beaten
- 2 cups creamed cottage cheese
- ¼ cup chopped onion
- 1 red bell pepper, diced
- 2 teaspoons dried parsley
- ½ teaspoon lemon peel
- 1 can salmon, drained

Dill Sauce:

- 1 ½ teaspoon butter
- 1 ½ teaspoon flour
- 1/8 teaspoon pepper
- 1 tablespoon lemon juice
- 1 ½ cup coffee creamer
- 2 teaspoons dried dill weed

Instructions:

- Beat the egg with the cream cheese and all the other filling ingredients in a bowl.
- Divide the filling in the pasta shells and place the shells in a 9x13 baking dish.
- Pour the coffee creamer around the stuffed shells then cover with a foil.
- Bake the shells for 30 minutes at 350 degrees F.
- Meanwhile, whisk all the ingredients for dill sauce in a saucepan.
- Stir for 5 minutes until it thickens.
- Pour this sauce over the baked pasta shells.
- Serve warm.

Nutritional information per serving:

Calories 268

Total Fat 4.8g

Saturated Fat 2g

Cholesterol 27mg

Sodium 86mg

Total Carbohydrate 42.6g

Dietary Fiber 2.1g

Sugars 2.4g

Protein 11.5g

Calcium 27mg

Phosphorous 314mg

Potassium 181mg

Herbed Vegetable Trout

Cooking time: 15 minutes

Servings: 4

Ingredients:

- 14 oz. trout fillets
- 1/2 teaspoon herb seasoning blend
- 1 lemon, sliced
- 2 green onions, sliced
- 1 stalk celery, chopped
- 1 medium carrot, julienne

Instructions:

- Prepare and preheat a charcoal grill over moderate heat.

- Place the trout fillets over a large piece of foil and drizzle herb seasoning on top.
- Spread the lemon slices, carrots, celery, and green onions over the fish.
- Cover the fish with foil and pack it.
- Place the packed fish in the grill and cook for 15 minutes.
- Once done, remove the foil from the fish.
- Serve.

Nutritional information per serving:

Calories 202

Total Fat 8.5g

Saturated Fat 1.5g

Cholesterol 73mg

Sodium 82mg

Carbohydrate 3.5g

Dietary Fiber 1.1g

Sugars 1.3g

Protein 26.9g

Calcium 70mg

Phosphorous 287mg

Potassium 560mg

Citrus Glazed Salmon

Cooking time: 17 minutes

Servings: 4

Ingredients:

- 2 garlic cloves, crushed
- 1 1/2 tablespoons lemon juice
- 2 tablespoons olive oil
- 1 tablespoon butter
- 1 tablespoon Dijon mustard
- 2 dashes cayenne pepper
- 1 teaspoon dried basil leaves
- 1 teaspoon dried dill
- 24 oz. salmon filet

Instructions:

- Place a 1-quart saucepan over moderate heat and add the oil, butter, garlic, lemon juice, mustard, cayenne pepper, dill, and basil to the pan.
- Stir this mixture for 5 minutes after it has boiled.
- Prepare and preheat a charcoal grill over moderate heat.
- Place the fish on a foil sheet and fold the edges to make a foil tray.
- Pour the prepared sauce over the fish.
- Place the fish in the foil in the preheated grill and cook for 12 minutes.
- Slice and serve.

Nutritional information per serving:

Calories 401

Total Fat 20.5g

Saturated Fat 5.3g

Cholesterol 144mg

Sodium 256mg

Carbohydrate 0.5g

Dietary Fiber 0.2g

Sugars 0.1g

Protein 48.4g

Calcium 549mg

Phosphorous 214mg

Potassium 446mg

Broiled Salmon Fillets

Cooking time: 13 minutes

Servings: 4

Ingredients:

- 1 tablespoon ginger root, grated
- 1 clove garlic, minced
- ¼ cup maple syrup
- 1 tablespoon hot pepper sauce
- 4 salmon fillets, skinless

Instructions:

- Grease a pan with cooking spray and place it over moderate heat.
- Add the ginger and garlic and sauté for 3 minutes then transfer to a bowl.
- Add the hot pepper sauce and maple syrup to the ginger-garlic.
- Mix well and keep this mixture aside.
- Place the salmon fillet in a suitable baking tray, greased with cooking oil.
- Brush the maple sauce over the fillets liberally
- Broil them for 10 minutes at the oven at broiler settings.
- Serve warm.

Nutritional information per serving:

Calories 289

Total Fat 11.1g

Saturated Fat 1.6g

Cholesterol 78mg

Sodium 80mg

Carbohydrate 13.6g

Dietary Fiber 0g

Sugars 11.8g

Protein 34.6g

Calcium 78mg

Phosphorous 230mg

Potassium 331mg

Crab Cakes

Cooking time: 20 minutes

Servings: 4

Ingredients:

- 1 lb. crab meat
- 1 egg
- 1/3 cup bell pepper, chopped
- 1/4 cup onion, chopped
- ¼ cup panko breadcrumbs
- 1/4 cup mayonnaise
- 1 tablespoon dry mustard
- 1 teaspoon black pepper
- 2 tablespoons lemon juice
- 1 tablespoon garlic powder
- dash cayenne pepper
- 3 tablespoons olive oil

Instructions:

- Mix the crab meat with all the spices, veggies, crackers, egg, and mayonnaise in a suitable bowl.

- Once it is well mixed, make 4 patties out of this mixture.
- Grease a suitable skillet and place it over moderate heat.
- Sear each Pattie for 5 minutes per side in the hot pan.
- Serve.

Nutritional information per serving:

Calories 315

Total Fat 20.4g

Saturated Fat 2.9g

Cholesterol 105mg

Sodium 844mg

Carbohydrate 13g

Dietary Fiber 1.3g

Sugars 3.3g

Protein 17.4g

Calcium 437mg

Phosphorous 288mg

Potassium 114mg

Broiled Shrimp

Cooking time: 5 minutes

Servings: 8

Ingredients:

- 1 lb. shrimp in shell

- 1/2 cup unsalted butter, melted
- 2 teaspoons lemon juice
- 2 tablespoons chopped onion
- 1 clove garlic, minced
- 1/8 teaspoon pepper

Instructions:

- Toss the shrimp with the butter, lemon juice, onion, garlic, and pepper in a bowl.
- Spread the seasoned shrimp in a baking tray.
- Broil for 5 minutes in an oven on broiler setting.
- Serve warm.

Nutritional information per serving:

Calories 164

Total Fat 12.8g

Saturated Fat 7.4g

Cholesterol 167mg

Sodium 242mg

Carbohydrate 0.6g

Dietary Fiber 0.1g

Sugars 0.2g

Protein 14.6g

Calcium 45mg

Phosphorous 215mg

Potassium 228mg

Grilled Lemony Cod

Cooking time: 10 minutes

Servings: 4

Ingredients:

- 1 lb. cod fillets
- 1 teaspoon salt-free lemon pepper seasoning
- 1/4 cup lemon juice

Instructions:

- Rub the cod fillets with lemon pepper seasoning and lemon juice.
- Grease a baking tray with cooking spray and place the salmon in the baking tray.
- Bake the fish for 10 minutes at 350 degrees F in a preheated oven.
- Serve warm.

Nutritional information per serving:

Calories 155

Total Fat 7.1g

Saturated Fat 1.1g

Cholesterol 50mg

Sodium 53mg

Carbohydrate 0.7g

Dietary Fiber 0.2g

Sugars 0.3g

Protein 22.2g

Calcium 43mg

Phosphorous 237mg

Potassium 461mg

Spiced Honey Salmon

Cooking time: 16 minutes

Servings: 4

Ingredients:

- 3 tablespoons honey
- 3/4 teaspoon lemon peel
- 1/2 teaspoon black pepper
- 1/2 teaspoon garlic powder
- 1 teaspoon water
- 16 oz. salmon fillets
- 2 tablespoons olive oil
- Dill, chopped, to serve

Instructions:

- Whisk the lemon peel with honey, garlic powder, hot water, and ground pepper in a small bowl.

- Rub this honey mixture over the salmon fillet liberally.
- Set a suitable skillet over moderate heat and add olive oil to heat.
- Set the spiced salmon fillets in the pan and sear them for 4 minutes per side.
- Garnish with dill.
- Serve warm.

Nutritional information per serving:

Calories 264

Total Fat 14.1g

Saturated Fat 2g

Cholesterol 50mg

Sodium 55mg

Carbohydrate 14g

Dietary Fiber 0.4g

Sugars 13.4g

Protein 22.5g

Calcium 67mg

Phosphorous 174mg

Potassium 507mg

CHAPTER 11:
Meat Recipes

Chicken Grapes Veronique

Cooking time: 17 minutes

Servings: 6

Ingredients:

- 6 chicken breasts, boneless, skinless
- 1/8 teaspoon ground nutmeg
- 4 teaspoons butter
- 2/3 cup white wine
- 2 tablespoons orange marmalade
- 3/4 teaspoon dried tarragon
- 2 teaspoons flour
- 1/2 cup half-and-half cream
- 1 1/2 cups grapes halved

Instructions:

- Set an 8-inch non-stick pan over moderate heat and add butter to melt.
- Sear the chicken in the melted butter until golden brown on both sides.
- Whisk the flour with cream and wine in a small bowl.

- Pour this slurry into the skillet over the chicken and mix well.
- Cook it on a simmer for 6 minutes.
- Add the marmalade, tarragon, and grapes.
- Cook for 1 minute and serve warm.

Nutritional information per serving:

Calories 231

Total Fat 6.5g

Saturated Fat 3.6g

Cholesterol 84mg

Sodium 87mg

Total Carbohydrate 9.4g

Dietary Fiber 0.2g

Sugars 6.7g

Protein 27.9g

Calcium 30mg

Phosphorous 387mg

Potassium 88mg

Maple Glazed Steak

Cooking time: 10 minutes

Servings: 4

Ingredients:

- 2 lbs. flank steak
- 1/4 teaspoon salt-free meat tenderizer
- ¼ teaspoon stevia
- 2 tablespoons lemon juice
- 2 tablespoons low sodium soy sauce
- 1 tablespoon maple syrup

Instructions:

- Pound the meat with a mallet then place it in a shallow dish.
- Drizzle the meat tenderizer over the meat.
- Whisk the rest of the ingredients and spread this marinade over the meat.
- Marinate the meat for 4 hours in the refrigerator.
- Bake the meat for 5 minutes per side at 350 degrees F.
- Slice and serve.

Nutritional information per serving:

Calories 471

Total Fat 18.9g

Saturated Fat 7.9g

Cholesterol 125mg

Sodium 385mg

Carbohydrate 2.1g

Dietary Fiber 0.1g

Sugars 1.6g

Protein 39.1g

Calcium 36mg

Phosphorous 280mg

Potassium 387mg

Sirloin Squash Medley

Cooking time: 9 minutes

Servings: 4

Ingredients:

- 8 oz. canned pineapple slices
- 2 garlic cloves, minced
- 2 teaspoons ginger root, minced
- 3 teaspoons olive oil
- 1 lb. sirloin tips
- 1 medium zucchini, diced
- 1 medium yellow squash, diced
- 1/2 medium red onion, diced

Instructions:

- Mix the pineapple juice with 1 teaspoon olive oil, ginger, and garlic in a Ziplock bag.
- Add the sirloin tips to the pineapple juice marinade and seal the bag.

- Place the bag in the refrigerator overnight.
- Switch on your gas oven and preheat at 450 degrees F.
- Layer 2 pans with a foil sheet and grease with 1 teaspoon olive oil.
- Spread the squash, onion, and pineapple rings in the prepared pans.
- Bake them for 5 minutes then transfer to the serving plate.
- Place the marinated sirloin tips on a baking sheet and bake for 4 minutes in the oven.
- Transfer the sirloin tips on top of the roasted vegetables.
- Serve.

Nutritional information per serving:

Calories 308

Total Fat 14.6g

Saturated Fat 4.5g

Cholesterol 65mg

Sodium 96mg

Carbohydrate 11.7g

Dietary Fiber 1.9g

Sugars 7.3g

Protein 28g

Calcium 31mg

Phosphorous 273mg

Potassium 496mg

Apple Chicken Curry

Cooking time: 1 hour 11 minutes

Servings: 8

Ingredients:

- 8 chicken breasts, skinless, boneless
- 1/4 teaspoon black pepper
- 2 apples, peeled, cored, and chopped
- 2 small onions, chopped
- 1 garlic clove, minced
- 3 tablespoons butter
- 1 tablespoon curry powder
- 1/2 tablespoon dried basil
- 3 tablespoons arrowroot powder
- 1 cup chicken broth
- 1 cup of rice milk

Instructions:

- Switch on your gas oven and preheat it at 350 degrees F.
- Set the chicken breasts in a baking pan and drizzle black pepper over them.
- Set a suitable saucepan over moderate heat and add the butter to melt.
- Add the onion, garlic, and apple, then sauté until soft.

- Stir in the basil and curry powder, then cook for 1 minute.
- Add the arrowroot and continue mixing for 1 minute.
- Stir in the rice milk and chicken broth then cook by stirring for 5 minutes.
- Pour this sauce over the chicken breasts in the baking pan.
- Bake the chicken for 60 minutes then serve.

Nutritional information per serving:

Calories 348

Total Fat 8g

Saturated Fat 2.8g

Cholesterol 141mg

Sodium 289mg

Carbohydrate 15.4g

Dietary Fiber 2.1g

Sugars 6.7g

Protein 25.3g

Calcium 55mg

Phosphorous 381mg

Potassium 139mg

Allspice Pulled Beef

Cooking time: 30 minutes

Servings: 12

Ingredients:

- 4 lbs. pot roast
- 2 cups water
- 3/4 cup ketchup
- 1/4 cup brown Swerve
- 1/3 cup vinegar
- 1/2 teaspoon allspice powder
- 1/4 cup onion

Instructions:

- Add the water and roast to a slow cooker and cover it.
- Cook for 10 hours on LOW setting then drain the roast while keeping 1 cup of its liquid.
- Transfer the cooked meat to a 9x13 inches pan and keep it aside.
- Whisk the resulting liquid, ketchup, vinegar, brown Swerve, minced onion, and allspice in a bowl.
- Add the beef meat to the marinade and mix well to coat, then marinate overnight in the refrigerator.
- Spread the marinade in a baking pan then bake for 30 minutes at 350 degrees F.
- Mix well and shred the baked beef with the help of two forks.

- Serve warm.

Nutritional information per serving:

Calories 313
Total Fat 21.5g
Saturated Fat 9.5g
Cholesterol 85mg
Sodium 221mg
Total Carbohydrate 5.9g
Dietary Fiber 0.1g
Sugars 3.5g
Protein 34.8g
Calcium 16mg
Phosphorous 107mg
Potassium 281mg

Zesty Steak Tacos

Cooking time: 20 minutes

Servings: 6

Ingredients:

- 1 (1 1/4 lb.) flank steak, trimmed
- 2 teaspoons lemon zest
- 3/4 teaspoon black pepper
- 2 tablespoons lemon juice

- 1 tablespoon olive oil
- 1 tablespoon lower-sodium soy sauce
- 3 garlic cloves, minced
- 12 (6-inch) corn tortillas
- 1 oz. feta cheese, crumbled

Instructions:

- Wrap the tortillas in a foil sheet and warm them for 10 minutes at 300 degrees F in the oven.
- Set a non-stick pan over moderate heat and add the oil to heat.
- Stir in the chicken, lemon juice, and seasoning.
- Cook for 5 minutes then add the peppers and onion.
- Stir and cook for 5 minutes until the chicken is tender.
- Garnish with cilantro.
- Serve with warmed tortillas and garnish with cheese.
- Enjoy.

Nutritional information per serving:

Calories 320
Total Fat 12g
Saturated Fat 4.1g
Cholesterol 54mg
Sodium 292mg
Carbohydrate 22.6g
Dietary Fiber 3.2g

Sugars 0.6g

Protein 32g

Calcium 58mg

Phosphorous 270mg

Potassium 432mg

Jamaican Drumsticks

Cooking time: 24 minutes

Servings: 10

Ingredients:

- 10 chicken drumsticks
- 1/3 cup olive oil
- 2 tablespoons brown Swerve
- 1 tablespoon dried thyme
- 2 teaspoons allspice, ground
- 2 teaspoons smoked paprika
- 1 teaspoon cinnamon
- 1 teaspoon ginger, ground
- 1 teaspoon cloves, ground
- 1 teaspoon cayenne pepper, ground
- 1/4 teaspoon black pepper

Instructions:

- Blend everything, except the chicken, in a blender until smooth.
- Mix the chicken with the blended mixture in a large Ziplock bag then seal it.
- Refrigerate the chicken drumsticks with its marinade for 24 hours.
- Prepare and preheat a grill over medium-high heat then grease the grill with cooking spray.
- Place the marinated chicken in the grill and grill for 12 minutes per side.
- Serve warm.

Nutritional information per serving:

Calories 148
Total Fat 9.5g
Saturated Fat 1.7g
Cholesterol 40mg
Sodium 39mg
Total Carbohydrate 1.4 g
Dietary Fiber 0.6g
Sugars 0.4g
Protein 13.8g
Calcium 19mg
Phosphorous 136mg
Potassium 120mg

Chicken with Asparagus

Cooking time: 17 minutes

Servings: 2

Ingredients:

- 8 oz. boneless, skinless chicken breast
- 2 1/2 tablespoons olive oil
- 1/2 teaspoon cracked black pepper
- 1/8 teaspoon cumin
- 1/8 teaspoon paprika
- 1/8 teaspoon chili powder
- 1/4 teaspoon crushed red pepper flakes
- 10 asparagus spears
- 1 ear corn on the cob
- 1/2 lemon
- 1 tablespoon chives

Instructions:

- Rub the chicken breast with olive oil, herb spice mix, red pepper flakes, and black pepper for seasoning.
- Set a suitable grill pan over moderate heat and grill the chicken for 6 minutes per side.
- Transfer the chicken to the serving plates.

- Now season the asparagus with black pepper and 2 teaspoons of olive oil.
- Grill the asparagus for 3 minutes per side then transfer it to the serving plates with the chicken.
- Rub the corn ear with 1 teaspoon olive oil and grill for 2 minutes per side.
- Transfer the corn ear to the serving plates and add lemon juice and chives on top.
- Serve.

Nutritional information per serving:

Calories 311

Total Fat 17.4g

Saturated Fat 2.1g

Cholesterol 73mg

Sodium 64mg

Carbohydrate 13.8g

Dietary Fiber 4.2g

Sugars 3.8g

Protein 28g

Calcium 45mg

Phosphorous 239mg

Potassium 785mg

Chicken Pineapple Curry

Cooking time: 3 hours 10 minutes

Servings: 6

Ingredients:

- 1 1/2 lbs. chicken thighs, boneless, skinless
- 1/2 teaspoon black pepper
- 1/2 teaspoon garlic powder
- 2 tablespoons olive oil
- 20 oz. canned pineapple
- 2 tablespoons brown Swerve
- 2 tablespoons soy sauce
- 1/2 teaspoon Tabasco sauce
- 2 tablespoons cornstarch
- 3 tablespoons water

Instructions:

- Begin by seasoning the chicken thighs with garlic powder and black pepper.
- Set a suitable skillet over medium-high heat and add the oil to heat.
- Add the boneless chicken to the skillet and cook for 3 minutes per side.
- Transfer this seared chicken to a Slow cooker, greased with cooking spray.
- Add 1 cup of the pineapple juice, Swerve, 1 cup of pineapple, tabasco sauce, and soy sauce to a slow cooker.

- Cover the chicken-pineapple mixture and cook for 3 hours on low heat.
- Transfer the chicken to the serving plates.
- Mix the cornstarch with water in a small bowl and pour it into the pineapple curry.
- Stir and cook this sauce for 2 minutes on high heat until it thickens.
- Pour this sauce over the chicken and garnish with green onions.
- Serve warm.

Nutritional information per serving:

Calories 256

Total Fat 10.4g

Saturated Fat 2.2g

Cholesterol 67mg

Sodium 371mg

Total Carbohydrate 13.6g

Dietary Fiber 1.5g

Sugars 8.4g

Protein 22.8g

Calcium 28mg

Phosphorous 107 mg

Potassium 308mg

Baked Pork Chops

Cooking time: 40 minutes

Servings: 6

Ingredients:

- 1/2 cup flour
- 1 large egg
- 1/4 cup water
- 3/4 cup breadcrumbs
- 6 (3 1/2 oz.) pork chops
- 2 tablespoons butter, unsalted
- 1 teaspoon paprika

Instructions:

- Begin by switching the oven to 350 degrees F to preheat.
- Mix and spread the flour in a shallow plate.
- Whisk the egg with water in another shallow bowl.
- Spread the breadcrumbs on a separate plate.
- Firstly, coat the pork with flour, then dip in the egg mix and then in the crumbs.
- Grease a baking sheet and place the chops in it.
- Drizzle the pepper on top and bake for 40 minutes.
- Serve.

Nutritional information per serving:

Calories 221

Total Fat 7.8g

Saturated Fat 1.9g

Cholesterol 93mg

Sodium 135mg

Carbohydrate 11.9g

Dietary Fiber 3.5g

Sugars 0.5g

Protein 24.7g

Calcium 13mg

Phosphorous 299mg

Potassium 391mg

Brisket Carrot Medley

Cooking time: 1 hour 45 minutes

Servings: 6

Ingredients:

- 1/2 medium onion, sliced
- 1 medium carrot, diced
- 2 1/2 lbs. beef brisket
- 2 teaspoons black pepper
- 2 tablespoons olive oil

- 3 bay leaves
- 2 cups reduced-sodium beef broth
- 3 cups of water
- 2 tablespoons vinegar

Instructions:

- Begin by switching the oven to 350 degrees F to preheat.
- Remove the fat and season the brisket with black pepper.
- Warm up the oil in a Dutch oven on medium-high heat.
- Sear the brisket for 5 minutes and flip to sear for another 5 minutes.
- Transfer this meat to a plate and add the carrots and onion to the pot.
- Cook by stirring for 4 minutes.
- Add the bay leaves and meat over the vegetables.
- Pour in the water, broth, and vinegar.
- Bring up to a boil then cook for 1.5 hours on medium-high heat until meat is tender.
- Slice the meat and serve with the gravy.

Nutritional information per serving:

Calories 335

Total Fat 14.2g

Saturated Fat 3.9g

Cholesterol 135mg

Sodium 114mg

Carbohydrate 2.8g

Dietary Fiber 0.8g

Sugars 1g

Protein 46.2g

Calcium 19mg

Phosphorous 197mg

Potassium 681mg

Beef Chili Rice

Cooking time: 15 minutes

Servings: 6

Ingredients:

- 2 tablespoons vegetable oil
- 1 lb. lean ground beef
- 1 cup onion, chopped
- 2 cups rice, cooked
- 1 ½ teaspoons chili con carne
- 1/8 teaspoon black pepper
- ½ teaspoon sage

Instructions:

- Add the oil, onion, and beef to a pot and cook, stirring until brown.

- Add the rice and other seasonings then mix well.
- Cover the beef rice mixture and remove it from the heat.
- Serve it after 10 minutes.
- Enjoy.

Nutritional information per serving:

Calories 484

Total Fat 11.7g

Saturated Fat 3.5g

Cholesterol 74mg

Sodium 361mg

Carbohydrate 38.2g

Dietary Fiber 4.5g

Sugars 0.9g

Protein 30.6g

Calcium 24mg

Phosphorous 248mg

Potassium 404mg

Beef Chili Chorizo

Cooking time: 10 minutes

Servings: 4

Ingredients:

- 3 garlic cloves, minced

- 1 lb. lean ground beef
- 2 tablespoons chili powder
- 2 teaspoons red or cayenne pepper
- 1 teaspoon black pepper
- 1 teaspoon ground oregano
- 2 teaspoons balsamic vinegar

Instructions:

- Begin by tossing all the ingredients into a bowl.
- Mix them thoroughly then spread the mixture in a baking pan.
- Bake the meat for 10 minutes at 325 degrees F in an oven.
- Slice and serve in crumbles.

Nutritional information per serving:

Calories 283

Total Fat 14.2g

Saturated Fat 5.4g

Cholesterol 96mg

Sodium 117mg

Carbohydrate 7.9g

Dietary Fiber 2.4g

Sugars 3.3g

Protein 30.9g

Calcium 43mg

Phosphorous 197mg

Potassium 585mg

Pork Fajitas

Cooking time: 8 minutes

Servings: 4

Ingredients:

- ½ green bell pepper, julienned
- ½ medium onion, julienned
- 1 garlic clove, minced
- ½ lb. lean, boneless pork, cut into strips
- ½ teaspoon dried oregano
- 1/4 teaspoon cumin
- 1 tablespoon pineapple juice
- 1 tablespoon vinegar
- 1/8 teaspoon hot pepper sauce
- ½ tablespoon olive oil
- 2 (8 inches) flour tortillas

Instructions:

- Begin by tossing the oregano, garlic, vinegar, cumin, hot sauce, and pineapple juice into a bowl.
- Place the pork in this marinade and mix well to coat, then refrigerate for 15 minutes.

- Meanwhile, you can preheat the oven at 325 degrees F.
- Wrap the tortillas in a foil and heat them in the oven for 2-3 minutes.
- Now heat a suitable griddle on moderate heat and add the pork strips, green peppers, oil, and onion.
- Cook well for 5 minutes until the pork is al dente.
- Serve warm in the warmed tortillas.

Nutritional information per serving:

Calories 385

Total Fat 13.5g

Saturated Fat 4.1g

Cholesterol 156mg

Sodium 102mg

Carbohydrate 8.7g

Dietary Fiber 1.4g

Sugars 1.9g

Protein 31g

Calcium 51mg

Phosphorous 238mg

Potassium 328mg

Apple Pork Loin

Cooking time: 40 minutes

Servings: 6

Ingredients:

- 2 tablespoons butter, unsalted
- 20 oz. apple pie filling
- 6 boneless pork loin chops
- Black pepper, to taste

Instructions:

- Switch on your gas oven and preheat it to 350 degrees F.
- Grease a 9x13 inches pan with cooking spray.
- Spread the apple pie filling in this prepared pan evenly.
- Top this layer with pork loin chops.
- Drizzle black pepper on top of the chops.
- Cover the pan with a foil sheet and bake for approximately 30 minutes.
- Remove the foil sheet and bake for another 10 minutes.
- Serve warm.

Nutritional information per serving:

Calories 389

Total Fat 9.2g

Saturated Fat 0.6g

Cholesterol 0mg

Sodium 534mg

Carbohydrate 45.1g

Dietary Fiber 4g

Sugars 15.1g

Protein 24.2g

Calcium 5mg

Phosphorous 250mg

Potassium 45mg

Caribbean Turkey Curry

Cooking time: 1 hour 30 minutes

Servings: 6

Ingredients:

- 1 1/2 lbs. turkey breast, with skin
- 2 tablespoons butter, melted
- 2 tablespoons honey
- ½ tablespoon mustard
- 1 teaspoon curry powder
- ½ teaspoon garlic powder

Instructions:

- Begin by placing the turkey breast in a shallow roasting pan.
- Insert the thermometer to monitor the temperature.
- Bake the turkey for 1.5 hours at 350 degrees F until its internal temperature reaches 170 degrees F.

- Meanwhile, thoroughly mix the honey, butter, curry powder, garlic powder, and mustard.
- Glaze the cooked turkey with this mixture liberally.
- Let it sit for 15 minutes for absorption.
- Slice and serve.

Nutritional information per serving:

Calories 237

Total Fat 9.1g

Saturated Fat 4.3g

Cholesterol 88mg

Sodium 1768mg

Carbohydrate 8.2g

Dietary Fiber 1.3g

Sugars 6.2g

Protein 31.6g

Calcium 25mg

Phosphorous 175mg

Potassium 537mg

Chicken Fajitas

Cooking time: 20 minutes

Servings: 8

Ingredients:

- 8 (6 inches) flour tortillas
- 1/4 cup green pepper, julienned
- 1/4 cup red pepper, julienned
- 1/2 cup onion, sliced
- 1/2 cup cilantro
- 2 tablespoons olive oil
- 12 oz. chicken breasts, boneless, cut into strips
- 1/4 teaspoon black pepper
- 2 teaspoon chili powder
- 1/2 teaspoon cumin
- 2 tablespoons lemon juice

Instructions:

- Begin by wrapping the tortillas in a foil.
- Warm them up for 10 minutes in a preheated oven at 300 degrees F.
- Now you can add the oil to a non-stick pan.
- Add the lemon juice, chicken and seasoning.
- Stir and cook for 5 minutes then add the onion and peppers.
- Continue cooking for 5 minutes approximately until the chicken is al dente.
- Stir in the cilantro, mix well and serve in the tortillas.

Nutritional information per serving:

Calories 173

Total Fat 7.5g

Saturated Fat 1.3g

Cholesterol 38mg

Sodium 56mg

Carbohydrate 12.4g

Dietary Fiber 2.1g

Sugars 0.9g

Protein 14g

Calcium 32mg

Phosphorous 209mg

Potassium 196mg

Hungarian Chicken Paprika

Cooking time: 1 hour 35 minutes

Servings: 6

Ingredients:

- 2 tablespoons olive oil
- 1/2 cup onion, chopped
- 1 tablespoon sweet Hungarian paprika
- 1/2 teaspoon black pepper
- 6 chicken breasts, diced
- 2 cups of water
- 1 cup reduced-fat sour cream

Instructions:

- Begin by greasing a large pan with olive oil.
- Add the onion and sauté until golden.
- Now you can add the pepper and paprika for seasoning,
- Place the chicken in the pan and sauté well for 5 minutes.
- Add water and then cover the chicken with a lid.
- Let it simmer for 1.5 hours on low heat.
- Stir in the sour cream and mix well.
- Serve warm and fresh.

Nutritional information per serving:

Calories 392

Total Fat 16g

Saturated Fat 6.4g

Cholesterol 157mg

Sodium 134mg

Carbohydrate 3.3g

Dietary Fiber 0.7g

Sugars 0.6g

Protein 35.1g

Calcium 52mg

Phosphorous 253mg

Potassium 99mg

Garlicky Balsamic Chicken

Cooking time: 30 minutes

Servings: 8

Ingredients:

- 2 cups low-sodium chicken broth
- 1/2 cup balsamic vinegar
- 1/2 cup white wine
- 1 tablespoon rosemary, chopped
- 8 chicken breasts, boneless, skinless
- 1 garlic head, chopped
- 2 tablespoons olive oil
- Black pepper, to taste

Instructions:

- Begin by mixing the wine, rosemary, broth, and vinegar in a 9x13 inch baking pan.
- Add the chicken breasts and rub well with the mixture. Marinate overnight.
- Grease a saucepan with oil and add the garlic.
- Sauté until golden, then keep the garlic aside.
- Season the marinated chicken with black pepper and sear it for 5 minutes per side until golden.
- Pour the reserved marinade over it along with the garlic.

- Cook on reduced heat for 15 minutes and flip the chicken after 7 minutes.
- Transfer the chicken to the serving plates.
- Cook the remaining cooking liquid until it thickens.
- Pour the sauce over the chicken.
- Serve warm and fresh.

Nutritional information per serving:

Calories 265

Total Fat 3.4g

Saturated Fat 0.1g

Cholesterol 130mg

Sodium 188mg

Carbohydrate 1.6g

Dietary Fiber 0.3g

Sugars 0.2g

Protein 37.3g

Calcium 11mg

Phosphorous 221mg

Potassium 34mg

Salisbury Meat Steak

Cooking time: 25 minutes

Servings: 4

Ingredients:

- 1 lb. steak, finely chopped
- 1 small onion, chopped
- ½ cup green pepper, chopped
- 1 teaspoon black pepper
- 1 egg
- 1 tablespoon olive oil
- ½ cup water
- 1 tablespoon corn starch

Instructions:

- Mix the steak with the green pepper, egg, black pepper and onion in a bowl.
- Add the oil to a skillet and place the patties in.
- Sear the steak patties for 5 minutes per side until golden brown.
- Add half of the water and let the patties simmer for 15 minutes.
- Whisk the remaining water with cornstarch in a bowl.
- Add this cornstarch mixture to the patties and cook until the sauce thickens.
- Serve warm.

Nutritional information per serving:

Calories 276

Total Fat 11.6g

Saturated Fat 3.7g

Cholesterol 142mg

Sodium 92mg

Carbohydrate 4.8g

Dietary Fiber 0.7g

Sugars 1.1g

Protein 33.1g

Calcium 16mg

Phosphorous 361mg

Potassium 524mg

CHAPTER 12:
Sauce Recipes

Alfredo Sauce

Cooking time: 5 minutes

Servings: 4

Ingredients:

- 4 oz. cream cheese
- 1/2 cup grated Parmesan cheese
- 3/4 cup low-fat milk
- 1/4 cup butter
- 1/4 teaspoon white pepper
- 1/8 teaspoon garlic powder

Instructions:

- Set a 2-quart saucepan over moderate heat and add the Parmesan cheese, cream cheese, butter, milk, garlic powder, and white pepper.
- Stir and cook this mixture for 5 minutes until the cheese is melted.
- Serve.

Nutritional information per serving:

Calories 311

Total Fat 27.8g

Saturated Fat 17.8g

Cholesterol 84mg

Sodium 446mg

Carbohydrate 4.2g

Dietary Fiber 0g

Sugars 2.5g

Protein 12.8g

Calcium 331mg

Phosphorous 43mg

Potassium 108mg

Barbeque Sauce

Cooking time: 20 minutes

Servings: 8

Ingredients:

- 1/3 cup corn oil
- ½ cup tomato juice
- 1 tablespoon brown Swerve
- 1 garlic clove
- 1 tablespoon paprika
- ¼ cup vinegar
- 1 teaspoon pepper

- 1/3 cup water
- ¼ teaspoon onion powder

Instructions:

- Toss all the ingredients into a suitable saucepan.
- Cook this sauce for 20 minutes with occasional stirring.
- Serve.

Nutritional information per serving:

Calories 93

Total Fat 9.2g

Saturated Fat 1.2g

Cholesterol 0mg

Sodium 42mg

Carbohydrate 0.5g

Dietary Fiber 0.5g

Sugars 0.2g

Protein 0.3g

Calcium 7mg

Phosphorous 31mg

Potassium 68mg

Apple Butter

Cooking time: 2 hours

Servings: 20

Ingredients:

- 4 1/2 cups apple sauce
- 2 cups granulated Swerve
- 1/4 cup vinegar
- 1/2 teaspoon ground cloves
- 1/2 teaspoon cinnamon

Instructions:

- Whisk the apple sauce, Swerve, vinegar, ground cloves, and cinnamon in a small roasting pan.
- Bake the mixture for 2 hours at 350 degrees F in a preheated oven until it thickens.
- Mix well and transfer to a mason jar.
- Serve.

Nutritional information per serving:

Calories 97

Total Fat 0g

Saturated Fat 0g

Cholesterol 0mg

Sodium 1mg

Carbohydrate 9.6g

Dietary Fiber 0.6g

Sugars 8.1g

Protein 0.1g

Calcium 3mg

Phosphorous 110mg

Potassium 40mg

Blackberry Sauce

Cooking time: 10 minutes

Servings: 10

Ingredients:

- 5 cups blackberries
- 1/2 tablespoon stevia
- 1 tablespoon arrowroot powder
- 1 tablespoon lemon juice
- 1 cup water

Instructions:

- Crush the berries in a saucepan and add the stevia and a cup of water.
- Bring the berries to a boil then lower the heat to a simmer.
- Whisk the arrowroot powder with 2 tablespoons of water in a bowl and add it to the berries.
- Stir and cook the berries for 1 minute until the sauce thickens.

- Remove the cooked berry sauce from heat and stir in lemon juice.
- Serve.

Nutritional information per serving:

Calories 60

Total Fat 0.4g

Saturated Fat 0g

Cholesterol 0mg

Sodium 1mg

Carbohydrate 14.8g

Dietary Fiber 3.1g

Sugars 10.5g

Protein 1g

Calcium 21mg

Phosphorous 72mg

Potassium 119mg

Blueberry Salsa

Cooking time: 0 minutes

Servings: 4

Ingredients:

- 1 cup blueberries
- 1 cup raspberries

- 1/4 cup red onion
- 2 tablespoons lime juice
- 1 tablespoon basil

Instructions:

- Add the berries, lime juice, onion, and basil to a food processor.
- Pulse until all the ingredients are finely chopped into a salsa.
- Serve.

Nutritional information per serving:

Calories 45

Total Fat 0.4g

Saturated Fat 0g

Cholesterol 0mg

Sodium 1mg

Carbohydrate 11.5g

Dietary Fiber 4.1g

Sugars 5.6g

Protein 0.8g

Calcium 14mg

Phosphorous 53mg

Potassium 112mg

Cranberry Salsa

Cooking time: 0 minutes

Servings: 4

Ingredients:

- 16 oz. canned whole cranberries, chopped
- 8 oz. canned pineapple, crushed
- 10 oz. frozen strawberries, chopped
- 1/2 cup apple sauce

Instructions:

- Toss the pineapple with the strawberries, cranberries, and apple sauce in a salad bowl.
- Refrigerate the salsa for 2 hours or until ready to use.
- Serve.

Nutritional information per serving:

Calories 127

Total Fat 0.1g

Saturated Fat 0g

Cholesterol 0mg

Sodium 2.3mg

Carbohydrate 29.3g

Dietary Fiber 6.7g

Sugars 17g

Protein 0.9g

Calcium 36mg

Phosphorous 61mg

Potassium 278mg

Strawberry Salsa

Cooking time: 0 minutes

Servings: 4

Ingredients:

- 1 1/2 cups strawberries
- 1/2 cup cucumber
- 1/2 cup red onion
- 2 tablespoons jalapeño pepper, halved and seeded
- 1 tablespoon mint
- 1 teaspoon lime rind
- 2 tablespoons lime juice
- 1 tablespoon orange juice
- 1 tablespoon honey

Instructions:

- Add the red onion, cucumber, strawberries, mint, and jalapeño to a food processor.

- Pulse until all the ingredients are chopped into a salsa.
- Add the lime juice, orange juice, honey, and mix well.
- Serve.

Nutritional information per serving:

Calories 49
Total Fat 0.2g
Saturated Fat 0g
Cholesterol 0mg
Sodium 3mg
Carbohydrate 13.2g
Dietary Fiber 1.9g
Sugars 8g
Protein 0.8g
Calcium 23mg
Phosphorous 113mg
Potassium 161mg

Garlic Sauce

Cooking time: 0 minutes

Servings: 6

Ingredients:

- 1 garlic head, cloves peeled
- 2 tablespoons lemon juice

- 1 cup olive oil

Instructions:

- Add the garlic and lemon juice to a blender and blend to puree the garlic.
- Slowly stir in the olive oil while blending the garlic mixture.
- Serve.

Nutritional information per serving:

Calories 290

Total Fat 33.6g

Saturated Fat 4.8g

Cholesterol 0mg

Sodium 1mg

Carbohydrate 0.7g

Dietary Fiber 0.1g

Sugars 0.2g

Protein 0.2g

Calcium 3mg

Phosphorous 20mg

Potassium 14mg

Cranberry Sauce

Cooking time: 10 minutes

Servings: 6

Ingredients:

- 1 cup granulated Swerve
- 12 oz. whole cranberries
- 1 cup water

Instructions:

- Set a 2-quart saucepan over medium-high heat and add the Swerve and 1 cup water.
- Bring the Swerve up to a boil, then add the cranberries and reduce the heat to a simmer.
- Cook, stirring gently for 10 minutes then pass the mixture through a fine sieve over a mixing bowl.
- Spread the berries in the sieve using the back of a spoon.
- Mix well the strained sauce.
- Serve.

Nutritional information per serving:

Calories 25
Total Fat 0g
Saturated Fat 0g
Cholesterol 0mg
Sodium 1mg
Carbohydrate 7g

Dietary Fiber 2.4g

Sugars 2.3g

Protein 0g

Calcium 4.4mg

Phosphorous 7mg

Potassium 44mg

Lemon Caper Sauce

Cooking time: 7 minutes

Servings: 6

Ingredients:

- 2 tablespoons butter, unsalted
- 1 1/2 teaspoon all-purpose flour
- 1/2 cup reduced-sodium chicken broth
- 1/4 cup white wine
- 2 tablespoons lemon juice
- 1 teaspoon capers
- 1/4 teaspoon white pepper

Instructions:

- Set a suitable skillet over low heat and add the butter to melt.
- Gradually stir in the flour and mix well for 1 minute.

- Pour in the broth and continue mixing for another 1 minute.
- Stir in the pepper, lemon juice, wine, capers, and lemon juice.
- Mix well and cook by stirring for 5 minutes until it thickens.
- Allow the sauce to cool down.
- Serve.

Nutritional information per serving:

Calories 48

Total Fat 4g

Saturated Fat 2.5g

Cholesterol 10mg

Sodium 107mg

Carbohydrate 0.9g

Dietary Fiber 0.1g

Sugars 0.3g

Protein 0.6g

Calcium 4mg

Phosphorous 63mg

Potassium 36mg

CHAPTER 13:
Dessert Recipes

Chocolate Trifle

Cooking time: 15 minutes

Servings: 4

Ingredients:

- 1 small plain sponge swiss roll
- 3 oz. custard powder
- 5 oz. hot water
- 16 oz. canned mandarins
- 3 tablespoons sherry
- 5 oz. double cream
- 4 chocolate squares, grated

Instructions:

- Whisk the custard powder with water in a bowl until dissolved.
- In a bowl, mix the custard well until it becomes creamy and let it sit for 15 minutes.
- Spread the swiss roll and cut it in 4 squares.
- Place the swiss roll in the 4 serving cups.

- Top the swiss roll with mandarin, custard, cream, and chocolate.
- Serve.

Nutritional information per serving:

Calories 315
Total Fat 13.5g
Saturated Fat 8.4g
Cholesterol 43mg
Sodium 185mg
Carbohydrate 40.1g
Dietary Fiber 1.4g
Sugars 9.1g
Protein 2.9g
Calcium 61mg
Phosphorous 184mg
Potassium 129mg

Pineapple Meringues

Cooking time: 0 minutes

Servings: 4

Ingredients:

- 4 meringue nests
- 8 oz. crème fraiche

- 2 oz. stem ginger, chopped
- 8 oz. can pineapple chunks

Instructions:

- Place the meringue nests on the serving plates.
- Whisk the ginger with crème Fraiche and pineapple chunks.
- Divide this the pineapple mixture over the meringue nests.
- Serve.

Nutritional information per serving:

Calories 312

Total Fat 22.8g

Saturated Fat 0g

Cholesterol 0mg

Sodium 41mg

Carbohydrate 25g

Dietary Fiber 0.7g

Sugars 23.1g

Protein 2.3g

Calcium 3mg

Phosphorous 104mg

Potassium 110mg

Baked Custard

Cooking time: 30 minutes

Servings: 1

Ingredients:

- 1/2 cup milk
- 1 egg, beaten
- 1/8 teaspoon nutmeg
- 1/8 teaspoon vanilla
- Sweetener, to taste
- 1/2 cup water

Instructions:

- Lightly warm up the milk in a pan, then whisk in the egg, nutmeg, vanilla and sweetener.
- Pour this custard mixture into a ramekin.
- Place the ramekin in a baking pan and pour ½ cup water into the pan.
- Bake the custard for 30 minutes at 325 degrees F.
- Serve fresh.

Nutritional information per serving:

Calories 127
Total Fat 7g

Saturated Fat 2.9g

Cholesterol 174mg

Sodium 119mg

Carbohydrate 6.6g

Dietary Fiber 0.1g

Sugars 6g

Protein 9.6g

Calcium 169mg

Phosphorous 309mg

Potassium 171mg

Strawberry Pie

Cooking time: 25 minutes

Servings: 6

Ingredients:

- 1 unbaked (9 inches) pie shell
- 4 cups strawberries, fresh
- 1 cup of brown Swerve
- 3 tablespoons arrowroot powder
- 2 tablespoons lemon juice
- 8 tablespoons whipped cream topping

Instructions:

- Spread the pie shell in the pie pan and bake it until golden brown.
- Now mash 2 cups of strawberries with the lemon juice, arrowroot powder, and Swerve in a bowl.
- Add the mixture to a saucepan and cook on moderate heat until it thickens.
- Allow the mixture to cool then spread it in the pie shell.
- Slice the remaining strawberries and spread them over the pie filling.
- Refrigerate for 1 hour then garnish with whipped cream.
- Serve fresh and enjoy.

Nutritional information per serving:

Calories 236

Total Fat 11.1g

Saturated Fat 3.3g

Cholesterol 3mg

Sodium 183mg

Carbohydrate 26g

Dietary Fiber 2.3g

Sugars 7.5g

Protein 2.2g

Calcium 23mg

Phosphorous 47.2mg

Potassium 178mg

Apple Crisp

Cooking time: 45 minutes

Servings: 6

Ingredients:

- 4 cups apples, peeled and chopped
- ½ teaspoon stevia
- 3 tablespoons brandy
- 2 teaspoons lemon juice
- 1/2 teaspoon cinnamon
- 1/8 teaspoon nutmeg
- 3/4 cup dry oats
- 1/4 cup brown Swerve
- 2 tablespoons flour
- 2 tablespoons butter

Instructions:

- Toss the oats with the flour, butter and brown Swerve in a bowl and keep it aside.
- Whisk the remaining crisp ingredients in an 8-inch baking pan.
- Spread the oats mixture over the crispy filling.
- Bake it for 45 minutes at 350 degrees F in a preheated oven.

- Slice and serve.

Nutritional information per serving:

Calories 214
Total Fat 4.8g
Saturated Fat 0.8g
Cholesterol 0mg
Sodium 48mg
Carbohydrate 26.2g
Dietary Fiber 4.8g
Sugars 15.7g
Protein 2.1g
Calcium 15mg
Phosphorous 348mg
Potassium 212mg

Almond Cookies

Cooking time: 12 minutes

Servings: 24

Ingredients:

- 1 cup butter, softened
- 1 cup granulate Swerve
- 1 egg
- 3 cups flour

- 1 teaspoon baking soda
- 1 teaspoon almond extract

Instructions:

- Beat the butter with the Swerve in a mixer then gradually stir in the remaining ingredients.
- Mix well until it forms a cookie dough then divide the dough into small balls.
- Spread each ball into ¾ inch rounds and place them in a cookie sheet.
- Poke 2-3 holes in each cookie then bake for 12 minutes at 400 degrees F.
- Serve.

Nutritional information per serving:

Calories 159

Total Fat 7.9g

Saturated Fat 1.3g

Cholesterol 7mg

Sodium 144mg

Carbohydrate 6.8g

Dietary Fiber 0.4g

Sugars 3.1g

Protein 1.9g

Calcium 6mg

Phosphorous 274mg

Potassium 23mg

Lime Pie

Cooking time: 5 minutes

Servings: 8

Ingredients:

- 5 tablespoons butter, unsalted
- 1 1/4 cups breadcrumbs
- 1/4 cup granulated Swerve
- 1/3 cup lime juice
- 14 oz. condensed milk
- 1 cup heavy whipping cream
- 1 (9 inches) pie shell

Instructions:

- Switch on your gas oven and preheat it to 350 degrees F.
- Whisk the cracker crumbs with the Swerve and melted butter in a suitable bowl.
- Spread this cracker crumbs crust in a 9 inches pie shell and bake it for 5 minutes.
- Meanwhile, mix the condensed milk with the lime juice in a bowl.
- Whisk the heavy cream in a mixer until foamy, then add in the condensed milk mixture.

- Mix well, then spread this filling in the baked crust.
- Refrigerate the pie for 4 hours.
- Slice and serve.

Nutritional information per serving:

Calories 391

Total Fat 22.4g

Saturated Fat 11.5g

Cholesterol 57mg

Sodium 252mg

Total Carbohydrate 32.9g

Dietary Fiber 0.3g

Sugars 27.4g

Protein 5.3g

Calcium 163mg

Phosphorous 199mg

Potassium 221mg

Buttery Lemon Squares

Cooking time: 35 minutes

Servings: 12

Ingredients:

- 1 cup refined Swerve
- 1 cup flour

- 1/2 cup butter, unsalted
- 1 cup granulated Swerve
- 1/2 teaspoon baking powder
- 2 eggs, beaten
- 4 tablespoons lemon juice
- 1 tablespoon butter, unsalted, softened
- 1 tablespoon lemon zest

Instructions:

- Start mixing ¼ cup refined Swerve, ½ cup butter, and flour in a bowl.
- Spread this crust mixture in an 8-inche square pan and press it.
- Bake this flour crust for 15 minutes at 350 degrees F.
- Meanwhile, prepare the filling by beating 2 tablespoons lemon juice, granulated Swerve, eggs, lemon rind, and baking powder in a mixer.
- Spread this filling in the baked crust and bake again for about 20 minutes.
- Meanwhile, prepare the squares' icing by beating 2 tablespoons lemon juice, 1 tablespoon butter, and ¾ cup refine Swerve.
- Once the lemon pie is baked well, allow it to cool.
- Sprinkle the icing mixture on top of the lemon pie then cut it into 36 squares.
- Serve.

Nutritional information per serving:

Calories 229

Total Fat 9.5g

Saturated Fat 5.8g

Cholesterol 50mg

Sodium 66mg

Carbohydrate 22.8g

Dietary Fiber 0.3g

Sugars 16g

Protein 2.1g

Calcium 18mg

Phosphorous 257mg

Potassium 51mg

Chocolate Gelatin Mousse

Cooking time: 5 minutes

Servings: 4

Ingredients:

- 1 teaspoon stevia
- 1/2 teaspoon gelatin
- 1/4 cup milk
- 1/2 cup chocolate chips
- 1 teaspoon vanilla

- 1/2 cup heavy cream, whipped

Instructions:

- Whisk the stevia with the gelatin and milk in a saucepan and cook up to a boil.
- Stir in the chocolate and vanilla then mix well until it has completely melted.
- Beat the cream in a mixer until fluffy then fold in the chocolate mixture.
- Mix it gently with a spatula then transfer to the serving bowl.
- Refrigerate the dessert for 4 hours.
- Serve.

Nutritional information per serving:

Calories 200

Total Fat 12.1g

Saturated Fat 8g

Cholesterol 27mg

Sodium 31mg

Carbohydrate 4.7g

Dietary Fiber 0.7g

Sugars 0.8g

Protein 3.2g

Calcium 68mg

Phosphorous 120mg

Potassium 100mg

Blackberry Cream Cheese Pie

Cooking time: 45 minutes

Servings: 8

Ingredients:

- 1/3 cup butter, unsalted
- 4 cups blackberries
- 1 teaspoon stevia
- 1 cup flour
- 1/2 teaspoon baking powder
- 3/4 cup cream cheese

Instructions:

- Switch your gas oven to 375 degrees F to preheat.
- Layer a 2-quart baking dish with melted butter.
- Mix the blackberries with stevia in a small bowl.
- Beat the remaining ingredients in a mixer until they form a smooth batter.
- Evenly spread this pie batter in the prepared baking dish and top it with blackberries.
- Bake the blackberry pie for about 45 minutes in the preheated oven.

- Slice and serve once chilled.

Nutritional information per serving:

Calories 239

Total Fat 8.4g

Saturated Fat 4.9g

Cholesterol 20mg

Sodium 63mg

Carbohydrate 26.2g

Dietary Fiber 4.5g

Sugars 15.1g

Protein 2.8g

Calcium 67mg

Phosphorous 105mg

Potassium 170mg

Apple Cinnamon Pie

Cooking time: 50 minutes

Servings: 12

Ingredients:

Apple Filling:

- 9 cups apples, peeled, cored and sliced
- 1 tablespoon stevia

- 1/3 cup all-purpose flour
- 2 tablespoons lemon juice
- 1 teaspoon ground cinnamon
- 2 tablespoons butter

Pie Dough:

- 2 1/4 cups all-purpose flour
- 1 teaspoon stevia
- 1 1/2 sticks unsalted butter
- 6 oz. cream cheese
- 3 tablespoons cold heavy whipping cream
- Water, if needed

Instructions:

- Start by preheating your gas oven at 425 degrees F.
- Mix the apple slices with cinnamon, 1 tablespoon of butter, lemon juice, flour and stevia in a bowl and keep it aside covered.
- Whisk the flour with stevia, butter, cream cheese and cream in mixing bowl to form the dough.
- If the dough is too dry, slowly add some water to make a smooth dough ball.
- Cut the dough into two equal-size pieces and spread them into a 9-inch sheet.
- Place one of the sheets at the bottom of a 9-inch pie pan.

- Evenly spread the apples in this pie shell and add a tablespoon of butter over it.
- Cover the apple filling with the second sheet of the dough and pinch down the edges.
- Make 1-inch deep cuts on top of the pie and bake for about 50 minutes until golden.
- Slice and serve.

Nutritional information per serving:

Calories 303

Total Fat 8.8g

Saturated Fat 5.3g

Cholesterol 26mg

Sodium 30mg

Carbohydrate 21.7g

Dietary Fiber 4.8g

Sugars 19.6g

Protein 4.2g

Calcium 21mg

Phosphorous 381mg

Potassium 229mg

Maple Crisp Bars

Cooking time: 5 minutes

Servings: 20

Ingredients:

- 1/3 cup butter
- 1 cup brown Swerve
- 1 teaspoon maple extract
- 1/2 cup maple syrup
- 8 cups puffed rice cereal

Instructions:

- Mix the butter with Swerve, maple extract, and syrup in a saucepan over moderate heat.
- Cook by slowly stirring this mixture for 5 minutes then toss in the rice cereal.
- Mix well, then press this cereal mixture in a 13x9 inches baking dish.
- Refrigerate the mixture for 2 hours then cut into 20 bars.
- Serve.

Nutritional information per serving:

Calories 107

Total Fat 3.1g

Saturated Fat 0.5g

Cholesterol 0mg

Sodium 36mg

Carbohydrate 10.6g

Dietary Fiber 0.1g

Sugars 5.4g

Protein 0.4g

Calcium 7mg

Phosphorous 233mg

Potassium 24mg

Pineapple Gelatin Pie

Cooking time: 5 minutes

Servings: 8

Ingredients:

- 2/3 cup graham cracker crumbs
- 2 1/2 tablespoons butter, melted
- 1 (20-oz) can crushed pineapple, juice packed
- 1 small gelatin pack
- 1 tablespoon lemon juice
- 2 egg whites, pasteurized
- 1/4 teaspoon cream of tartar

Instructions:

- Whisk the crumbs with the butter in a bowl then spread them onto an 8-inch pie plate.
- Bake the crust for 5 minutes at 425 degrees F.
- Meanwhile, mix the pineapple juice with the gelatin in a saucepan.

- Place it over low heat then add the pineapple and lemon juice. Mix well.
- Beat the cream of tartar and egg whites in a mixer until creamy.
- Add the cooked pineapple mixture then mix well.
- Spread this filling in the baked crust.
- Refrigerate the pie for 4 hours then slice.
- Serve.

Nutritional information per serving:

Calories 106

Total Fat 4.2g

Saturated Fat 0.6g

Cholesterol 0mg

Sodium 117mg

Carbohydrate 14.5g

Dietary Fiber 0.5g

Sugars 9.4g

Protein 2.2g

Calcium 3mg

Phosphorous 231mg

Potassium 33mg

Cherry Pie Dessert

Cooking time: 40 minutes

Servings: 8

Ingredients:

- 1/2 cup butter, unsalted
- 2 eggs
- 1 cup granulated Swerve
- 1 cup sour cream
- 1 teaspoon vanilla
- 2 cups all-purpose flour
- 1 teaspoon baking powder
- 1 teaspoon baking soda
- 20 oz. cherry pie filling

Instructions:

- First, begin by setting your gas oven at 350 degrees F.
- Soften the butter first, then beat it with the cream eggs, Swerve, vanilla, and sour cream in a mixer.
- Separately mix the flour with the baking soda and baking powder.
- Add this mixture to the egg mixture and mix well until smooth.
- Spread the batter evenly in a 9x13 inch baking pan.
- Bake the pie for 40 minutes in the oven until golden from the surface.
- Slice and serve with cherry pie filling on top.

Nutritional information per serving:

Calories 470

Total Fat 19g

Saturated Fat 11.4g

Cholesterol 84mg

Sodium 285mg

Carbohydrate 43.2g

Dietary Fiber 1.3g

Sugars 14.9g

Protein 5.9g

Calcium 82mg

Phosphorous 249mg

Potassium 232mg

Strawberry Pizza

Cooking time: 15 minutes

Servings: 12

Ingredients:

- Crust:
- 1 cup flour
- 1/4 cup Swerve
- 1/2 cup butter

Filling:

- 8 oz. cream cheese, softened
- 1/2 teaspoon vanilla
- ¾ tablespoon stevia
- 2 cups sliced strawberries

Instructions:

- Mix the flour with the Swerve, butter, and enough water to make a dough.
- Spread this dough evenly in a pie pan.
- Bake the crust for 15 minutes at 350 degrees F.
- Beat the cream cheese with the stevia and vanilla in a mixer until fluffy.
- Spread this cream cheese filling in the crust and top it with strawberries.
- Serve.

Nutritional information per serving:

Calories 235

Total Fat 14.5g

Saturated Fat 9g

Cholesterol 41mg

Sodium 112mg

Carbohydrate 12.8g

Dietary Fiber 1g

Sugars 9.3g

Protein 2.8g

Calcium 25mg

Phosphorous 236mg

Potassium 84mg

Pumpkin Cinnamon Roll

Cooking time: 15 minutes

Servings: 24

Ingredients:

Dough:

- 1 1/2 cups milk
- 1/2 cup olive oil
- 1/2 cup granulated Swerve
- 2 1/4 teaspoons active dry yeast
- 1 cup pumpkin puree
- 4 1/2 cups flour
- 1/2 teaspoon ground cinnamon
- 1/4 teaspoon ground ginger
- 1/4 teaspoon ground nutmeg
- 1/2 teaspoon baking powder
- 1/2 teaspoon baking soda
- Melted butter, for buttering pans

Filling:

- 1/2 cup butter, melted
- 1/2 cup brown Swerve
- 1/2 cup granulated Swerve
- 1/2 teaspoon cinnamon
- 1/2 teaspoon ground ginger
- 1/4 teaspoon ground nutmeg

Instructions:

- Switch on your gas oven and let it preheat at 375 degrees F.
- Whisk all the ingredients for the dough in a mixing bowl.
- Spread the dough in a loaf pan into a ½-inch layer and bake it for 15 minutes.
- Meanwhile, whisk all the ingredients for the filling in a bowl.
- Place the baked cake in a serving plate and top it with the prepared filling.
- Roll the cake and slice it.
- Serve.

Nutritional information per serving:

Calories 201
Total Fat 9.2g
Saturated Fat 3.7g
Cholesterol 12mg
Sodium 63mg

Carbohydrate 14.9g

Dietary Fiber 1g

Sugars 3.1g

Protein 3.2g

Calcium 32mg

Phosphorous 277mg

Potassium 91mg

Peppermint Cookies

Cooking time: 12 minutes

Servings: 12

Ingredients:

- 2 1/2 cups all-purpose flour
- 1 teaspoon baking soda
- 3/4 cup cocoa powder
- 1 cup butter, unsalted
- 1 cup granulated Swerve
- 1 cup brown Swerve
- 2 large eggs
- 1 teaspoon vanilla extract
- 1/2 teaspoon peppermint extract
- 1 cup of chocolate chips
- 1 cup peppermint crunch pieces
- 1/2 cup crushed candies

Instructions:

- Begin by softening the butter at room temperature.
- Add 12 peppermint candies to a Ziplock bag and crush them using a mallet.
- Beat the butter with the egg, Swerve, and peppermint extract in a mixer until fluffy.
- Stir in the baking powder and flour and mix well until smooth.
- Stir in the crushed peppermint candies and refrigerate the dough for 1 hour.
- Meanwhile, you can layer a baking sheet with parchment paper.
- Switch the oven to 350 degrees F to preheat.
- Now crush the remaining candies and keep them aside.
- Make ¾ inch balls out of the dough and place them in the baking sheet.
- Drizzle the crushed candies over the balls.
- Bake them for 12 minutes until slightly browned.
- Serve fresh and enjoy.

Nutritional information per serving:

Calories 362

Total Fat 16.5g

Saturated Fat 10.1g

Cholesterol 71mg

Sodium 224mg

Carbohydrate 31.7g

Dietary Fiber 2.5g

Sugars 16.9g

Protein 5.8g

Calcium 25mg

Phosphorous 233mg

Potassium 138mg

Pumpkin Cheese Pie

Cooking time: 6 minutes

Servings: 8

Ingredients:

- 1 1/4 cups graham cracker crumbs
- 1/3 cup unsalted butter, melted

Filling:

- 8 oz. cream cheese, softened
- 1/2 cup pumpkin
- 1 teaspoon stevia
- 2 eggs
- 1 teaspoon vanilla
- 1 teaspoon cinnamon
- 1/2 teaspoon nutmeg

Sauce:

- 1 cup water
- 1 tablespoon cornstarch
- 2 teaspoons lemon juice
- 2 cups fresh cranberries

Instructions:

- Blend the cracker crumbs with the butter in a bowl then spread them onto a 9-inch pie plate.
- Beat the cream cheese with the pumpkin, stevia, egg, cinnamon, nutmeg, vanilla in a mixer.
- Whisk the water with the lemon juice and cranberries in a saucepan, then cook, stirring slowly until it thickens.
- Spread the cream cheese filling in the crumbs crust then top it with cranberries sauce.
- Refrigerate the pie for 4 hours.
- Slice and serve.

Nutritional information per serving:

Calories 268

Total Fat 19.8g

Saturated Fat 7.8g

Cholesterol 72mg

Sodium 307mg

Carbohydrate 7g

Dietary Fiber 2.4g

Sugars 2.1g

Protein 4.6g

Calcium 44mg

Phosphorous 371mg

Potassium 135mg

Ribbon Cakes

Cooking time: 20 minutes

Servings: 21

Ingredients:

- 1 ½ cups flour
- ½ cup of Swerve
- ½ teaspoon baking powder
- ½ cup butter, softened
- 1 whole eggs
- ½ egg white
- ¼ teaspoon vanilla
- ½ cup jelly
- 1 tablespoon brown Swerve

Instructions:

- Prepare and preheat the oven at 375 degrees F.

- Whisk the flour with the baking powder and Swerve in a bowl.
- Beat the butter with cornmeal, eggs, egg white, and vanilla in a beater.
- Stir in the flour and mix well to form a dough.
- Knead this dough on a floured surface and cut it into 2 equal pieces.
- Spread each piece into a 1/8-inch thick sheet.
- Spread one dough layer in an 11x15 inch cookie pan and top it with jelly.
- Slice the second layer into ½-inch wide strips.
- Place these strips over the jelly and arrange them in a crisscross manner.
- Drizzle brown Swerve over the dough then bake for 20 minutes approximately.
- Cut the baked pie into 1x2 inches rectangles.
- Serve.

Nutritional information per serving:

Calories 94

Total Fat 4.7g

Saturated Fat 2.9g

Cholesterol 19mg

Sodium 17mg

Carbohydrate 13.6g

Dietary Fiber 0.3g

Sugars 2.7g

Protein 1.3g

Calcium 10mg

Phosphorous 37mg

Potassium 21mg

Pineapple Pudding

Cooking time: 15 minutes

Servings: 12

Ingredients:

- 3 tablespoons all-purpose flour
- 1 tablespoon brown Swerve
- 4 large eggs
- 1 cup milk
- 1 cup water
- 1 teaspoon vanilla extract
- 2 cups pineapple chunks, drained
- 2 drops liquid stevia
- 30 vanilla wafers

Instructions:

- Prepare and preheat the oven at 425 degrees F.

- Whisk the flour with 1 whole egg, 3 egg yolks, and Swerve in a bowl.
- Place this bowl over boiling water and stir in the vanilla essence, stevia, milk and water.
- Stir and cook this mixture until it thickens.
- Remove the custard from the heat and spread it in a 1 ½ quart casserole dish.
- Top the custard with half of the vanilla wafers and half of the pineapple.
- Repeat the layers in the same manner.
- Beat the egg whites with the Swerve in an electric mixer until fluffy.
- Top the custard casserole with egg white fluff.
- Bake this custard casserole for 5 minutes in the oven.
- Serve.

Nutritional information per serving:

Calories 139
Total Fat 3.4g
Saturated Fat 1.1g
Cholesterol 68mg
Sodium 60mg
Carbohydrate 15.3g
Dietary Fiber 0.6g
Sugars 7.4g
Protein 3.5g

Calcium 41mg

Phosphorous 309mg

Potassium 75mg

CONCLUSION

In a nutshell, the purpose of the Renal Diet is to provide a healthy lifestyle and dietary approach to keep the kidneys healthy and functioning. All it takes is some precautionary measures and added attention to the type of ingredients we consume to protect our precious blood-filtering kidneys. Remember, there is no external treatment good enough to alter the functions of our natural body organs. It is, therefore, essential to opt for a lifestyle that can prevent chronic kidney diseases. In this cookbook, the author has managed to unveil the true harms of the kidney disease for the readers, so that everyone can take the necessary steps towards a healthier life. The entire recipes section is full of a variety of flavorsome recipes for different times of the day. Add this variety to your Renal diet and make your meals exciting again.

CPSIA information can be obtained
at www.ICGtesting.com
Printed in the USA
BVHW092100011220
594609BV00007B/683